The Slim Drinker
Kate Clarke

The Slim Drinker

LOW on calories

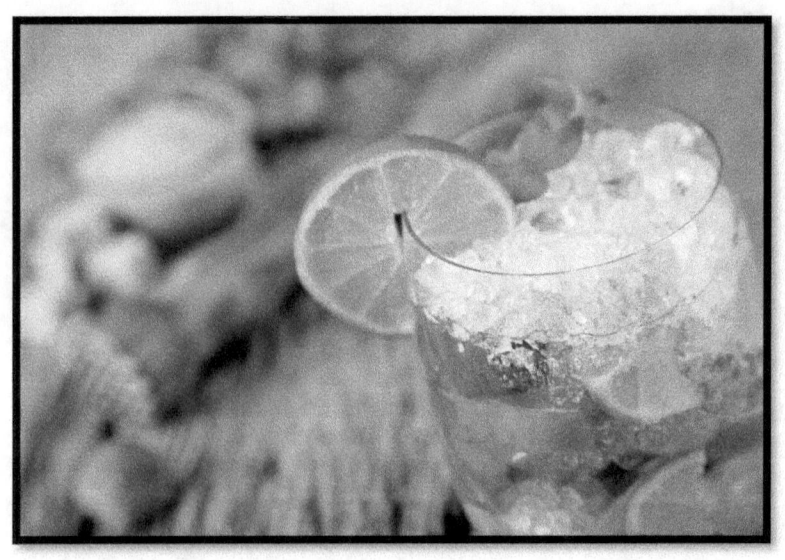

BIG on fun

Published by ROC Publishing 2015

Copyright and Trademarks

This publication is Copyright 2015 by **ROC Publishing**. All products, publications, software and services mentioned and recommended in this publication are protected by trademarks. In such instance, all trademarks & copyright belong to the respective owners. All rights reserved. No part of this book may be reproduced or transferred in any form or by any means, graphic, electronic, or mechanical including photocopying, recording, taping, or by any information storage retrieval system, without the written permission of the author. Pictures used in this book are either royalty free pictures bought from stock-photo websites or have the source mentioned underneath the picture.

Disclaimer and Legal Notice

This product is not legal or medical advice and should not be interpreted in that manner. You need to do your own due-diligence to determine if the content of this product is right for you. The author and the affiliates of this product are not liable for any damages or losses associated with the content of this product. While every attempt has been made to verify the information shared in this publication, neither the author nor the affiliates assume any responsibility for errors, omissions or contrary interpretation of the subject matter herein. Any perceived slights to any specific person(s) or organization(s) are purely unintentional. We have no control over the nature, content and availability of the web sites listed in this book. The inclusion of any website links does not necessarily imply a recommendation or endorse the views expressed within them. ROC Publishing takes no responsibility for, and will not be liable for, the websites being temporarily unavailable or being removed from the Internet.The accuracy and completeness of information provided herein are not guaranteed or warranted to produce any particular results, and the advice and strategies, contained herein may not be suitable for every individual. The author shall not be liable for any loss incurred as a consequence of the use and application, directly or indirectly, of any information presented in this work.The publication is designed to provide information in regards to the subject matter covered.

Foreword

For many people, an alcoholic beverage or two is the perfect way to unwind after a long and stressful day. Enjoying the occasional drink is by no means a bad thing but, if you are trying to lose weight or get fit, it could put a damper on your plans. The key to achieving your goals without giving up the buzz you crave is to find alcoholic beverages that are low in calories but high in alcohol content – these drinks will give you the best bang for your buzz.

In this book you will find a wealth of information to help you understand how alcohol affects your body and what you can do to maximize your buzz without having to add another notch to your belt. You will receive tricks for planning your nights of drinking and for selecting the right drinks. You will also receive a collection of delicious and buzz-worthy drinks that won't tip the scales or set you back from achieving your goals.

Acknowledgements

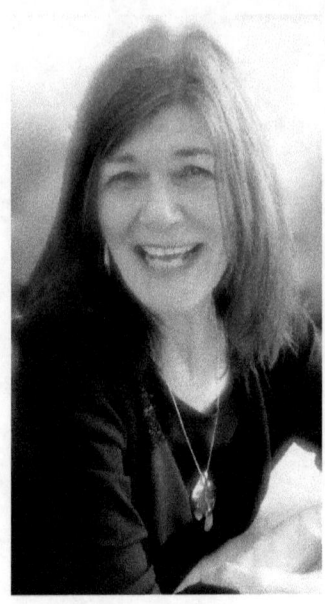

I would like to extend my sincerest thanks to all my family for supporting me throughout the journey of writing this book.

I love you all.

Special thanks to my niece, Zoë. Who so graciously volunteered to taste-test the recipes I concocted. It's been great fun.

I hope you enjoy the book as much as I've enjoyed writing it and I wish you exciting times in your 'Slim Drinking' challenges.

TABLE OF CONTENTS

CHAPTER ONE: INTRODUCTION	1
CHAPTER TWO: DETERMINING YOUR GOALS	3
1.) Understanding Alcohol Content	4
a.) What Are Your Goals?	6
2.) The Best Bang for Your Buzz	9
1.) Calorie-Dense Drinks	10
2.) Low-Calorie, High Alcohol Drinks	12
CHAPTER THREE: ALCOHOL'S EFFECTS ON THE BODY	15
1.) Understanding the Effects of Alcohol	16
2.) Alcohol and Fat Storage – Beer Belly	20
a.) What Causes Beer Belly?	22
b.) The Dangers of Abdominal Obesity	23
c.) Gluten Sensitivity	25
d.) Best Beers to Drink	29
3.) Water and Alcohol	31
a.) Water and Your Health	32
b.) Staying Hydrated While Drinking	33
c.) Rehydrating the Day After	34
4.) Sleep and Alcohol	35
5.) Short and Long-Term Effects	37
CHAPTER FOUR: FACTORS THAT EFFECT INTOXICATION	41

1.) Alcohol and Food	42
2.) Body Weight and Type	44
3.) Rate of Consumption/Strength of Drink	45
4.) Other Factors	47

CHAPTER FIVE: MAKING A PLAN FOR DRINKING — 49

1.) Before You Drink	50
2.) Before You Drink	52
3.) The Day After	54
a.) Day-After Juice and Smoothie Recipes	56
Ginger, Carrot, Beet Juice	57
Protein-Packed Spinach Smoothie	58
Lemon Dandelion Green Juice	59
Detoxifying Coconut Smoothie	60
Savory Tomato Cucumber Juice	61
Chocolate Almond Banana Smoothie	62
Celery Apple Juice with Lime	63
Blueberry Chia Seed Smoothie	64
4.) Taking a Break	65

CHAPTER SIX: HIGHEST AND LOWEST CALORIE DRINKS — 67

1.) Highest Calorie Cocktails	68
2.) Lowest Calorie Cocktails	69

CHAPTER SEVEN: HEALTHY/LOW-CALORIE COCKTAIL CHOICES — 71

1.) Cocktails Under 200 Calories	72
Raspberry Cosmo on Ice	73

Gin and Tonic - Light	74
Mulled Cider for a Group	75
Cucumber Honey Cocktail	77
Hot Toddy	78
Extra-Light Margarita	79
Fresh Mint Mojito	80
Mulled Wine for a Crowd	81
Refreshing Sea Breeze	82
Vanilla Cake Cocktail	83
Tequila Soda with Lime	84
Sour Apple Martini	85
2.) Healthy Cocktails with Fruit	**86**
Frozen Blueberry Margarita	87
Sweet Tropical Limeade	88
Gin and Watermelon Fizz	89
Refreshing Blueberry Bellini	90
Blackberry Coconut Daiquiri	91
Bloody Mary	92
Raspberry Mojito	93
Strawberry Coconut Margarita	94
Razzy Pink Cosmo	95
Orange Old Fashioned	96
Kiwi Tom Collins	97
Tropical Pineapple Champagne Cooler	98
Spicy Grapefruit Margarita	99
Lemon Gin Fizz with Rosemary	100
Watermelon Sunrise	101
Honeydew Sparklers	102
Melon Sangria	103
Mint Strawberry Mojito	104

RESOURCES   105

INDEX   110

Chapter One: Introduction

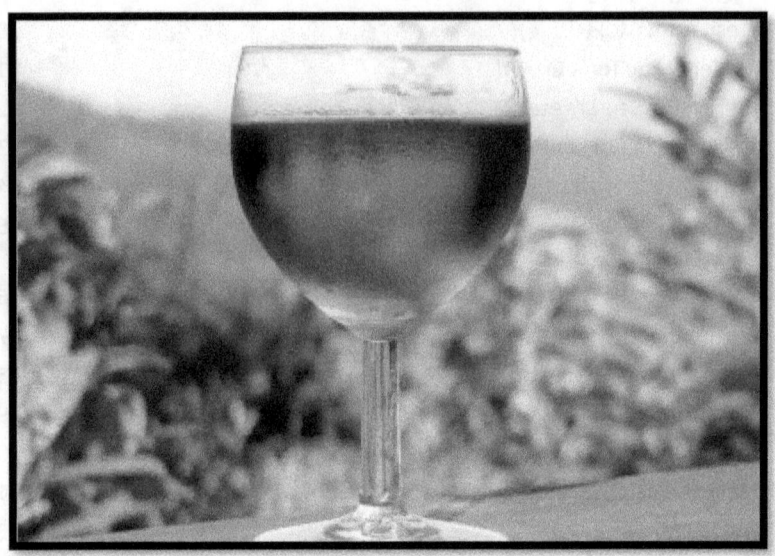

After a long day at the office or a hectic afternoon of ferrying the kids to soccer practice and ballet, you probably feel like you could use a drink. Enjoying an alcoholic beverage or two is a very common way to unwind and relax, to let go of the stress of our everyday lives. While drinking a cold beer or a glass of wine might make you feel better, it may be interfering with your goals of looking better. Many alcoholic beverages are high in carbs and calories which can significantly increase your daily caloric intake which could lead to weight gain.

Chapter One: Introduction

If you want to lose weight, get fit, or simply look better, you may be wondering whether alcohol has a place in your healthy routine. While overindulging in alcoholic beverages is never healthy, having the occasional drink is unlikely to do you any harm. What you have to be mindful of, however, is how your drinking aligns with your health and weight loss goals. If you are trying to lose weight, you need to be conscious of the calorie content of your drinks and you need to make sure that drinking them doesn't put you over your daily calorie goal.

In this book you will receive all of the information you need to "drink and shrink" – that is, tips and tricks for finding the right drinks to give you the buzz you crave without causing you to add another notch to your belt. Here you will find valuable information about the effects of alcohol on the body and tips for planning when and what you will drink while still achieving your goals. You will also receive a collection of low-calorie drink recipes to help you get your buzz on without tipping the scales. So what are you waiting for? Get to reading!

Chapter Two: Determining Your Goals

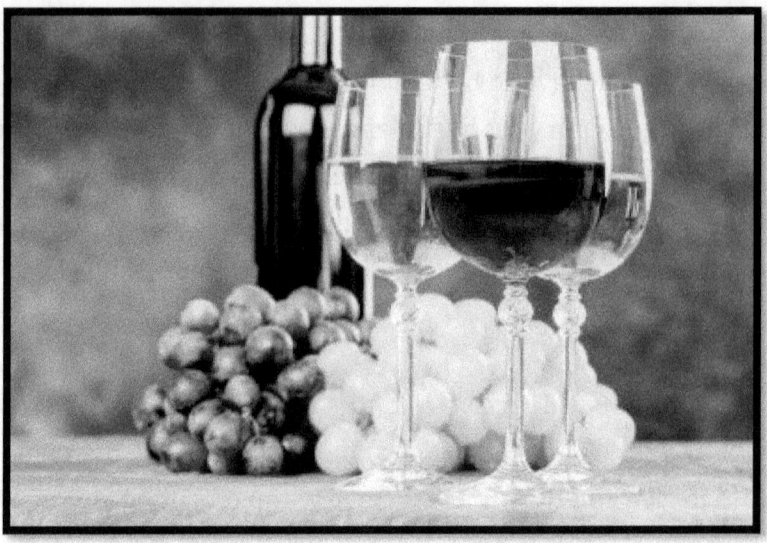

If you are concerned about the calorie content of alcoholic beverages it is probably because you are trying to lose weight. The key to weight loss is to consume fewer calories than you burn on a daily basis and that includes the calories your drink. Many people do not realize that some of the most popular alcoholic drinks are very high in calories and that overindulging in those drinks could be sabotaging their weight loss. If you want to continue to enjoy alcoholic beverages while still meeting your health or weight loss goals, you need to learn how to achieve your desired level of buzz with the fewest number of calories possible. To do this you need to understand alcohol content and its effects on your body.

Chapter Two: Determining Your Goals

1.) *Understanding Alcohol Content*

Whether you are trying to lose weight, improve your health, or get fit, you need to be intentional about which drinks you choose. Dark beers, IPAs and dessert wines are high in calories and those calories can add up quickly during a night of drinking. On the flip side, sparking wine and distilled liquors are some of the drinks with the lowest number of calories per serving while still giving you a good buzz. Before we get into the best drinks for your buzz, however, you should take the time to learn about the alcohol content of your favorite drinks and how it is measured. Having this knowledge will help you to determine which drinks are the best for your buzz.

When you look at a bottle of distilled liquor at the liquor store, you will see the word "proof" paired with a number – this tells you how much alcohol the liquor actually contains. During the early 1700s, the "proof" of distilled liquors was tested by adding gunpowder and setting the liquor on fire. If the liquor did not burn, the alcohol content was too low – if it burned too quickly it was too high. When he flames glowed a steady blue, the proof was just right – this typically equated to 100 proof, or about 57.15% ethanol by volume.

Today, proof is calculated by doubling the percentage of alcohol that is found in the solution kept at 60°F (15.6°C). Using this calculation, 100 proof liquor contains about 50% alcohol and 150

Chapter Two: Determining Your Goals

proof liquor contains about 75%. Proof measurements vary slightly from one country to another but the alcohol content of standard drinks like wine, beer, and liquor are roughly the same.

Consult the chart below to determine the alcohol content of different proofs of liquor:

Alcohol Content by Proof	
Proof	Alcohol Content
100 proof	50%
80 proof	40%
40 proof	20%
30 proof	15%
20 proof	10%

Another way to measure the alcohol content of a beverage is by volume, or ABV. The ABV of a given beverage is a measure of the ethanol content given a certain volume of beverage – the ABV is expressed as a volume percent. Alcohol by volume is calculated by measuring the number of milliliters ethanol contained in a 100 milliliters of solution at 20°C (68°F). Table wine typically has an ABV between 8 and 14% while regular beer has a much lower ABV around 4 to 6%. The lower the ABV of a beverage, the more you need to drink to feel a buzz. The more you drink, the more calories you consume, and the further you find yourself from achieving your goals.

Chapter Two: Determining Your Goals

The chart below lists the average ABV of popular alcoholic beverages for your reference:

ABV of Popular Drinks	
Drink	**Average ABV**
Regular Beer	2% - 12% (avg. 4-6%)
Malt Liquor	5%
Strong Ale	8% - 15%
Wine	9% - 16% (avg. 12.5-14.5%)
Dessert Wine	14% - 25%
Sake	15% (18%-20% undiluted)
Liqueur (flavored)	15% - 55%
Tequila	32% - 60%
Vodka	35% - 60%
Brandy	35% - 60%
Rum	37.5% - 80%
Gin	40% - 50%
Whisky	40% - 68%

a.) What Are Your Goals?

Now that you understand the basics about how alcohol content is measured you can connect that information to your goals in order to determine your drinking strategy. So what are your goals? Do you want to lose weight and lower your body fatpercentage? Are you trying to build muscle and improve your body image? Do you have a tendency to overindulge in alcohol

Chapter Two: Determining Your Goals

and want to get your drinking under control? <u>Below you will find tips related to each of these goals</u>:

Lose Weight/Lower Body Fat Percentage

Losing weight and lowering your body fat percentage go hand in hand, but how to you accomplish that goal? You need to reduce your daily calorie intake so it is less than the number of calories your body burns on a daily basis. To accomplish this you need to limit your carbs and calories. Ideally, you should limit your drinking as much as possible but, if you still want to drink on occasion, you should select low-calorie, high ABV drinks.

Build More Muscle

In order to build muscle you need to consume a lot of protein and that is something you won't find in a glass of wine or a bottle of beer. If you pair the occasional drink with a healthy lifestyle and strength training regimen you can still meet your goals. Just be careful about overindulging in high-carb and high-calorie beverage like beer.

Look Better and Feel Better About Yourself

If you simply want to look better and feel better about yourself, alcohol is not the solution. Take better care of yourself by following a healthy diet, engaging in regular exercise, and getting plenty of sleep. If you are able to maintain these healthy habits

Chapter Two: Determining Your Goals

while still enjoying the occasional drink, good for you! If you hit a plateau, however, and see a stall in your results then you might want to stop drinking for a little while until you get back on track.

Get Your Drinking Under Control

If you have a problem controlling yourself with alcohol – if one or two drinks quickly turns into seven or eight – your best bet is to stay away from drinking. Find a non-alcoholic beverage you like and order that when you go out with friends. You might even consider volunteering to be the designated driver so you have a valid reason for why you aren't drinking if your friends ask.

Now that you've determined your goals you can start to think about how alcohol fits into your plan. In the following sections you will receive information about low-calorie, high-ABV drinks that can help you achieve your desired level of buzz without getting you off track with your goals. Just remember to drink responsibly and to pace yourself until you know how your body reacts to certain drinks.

Chapter Two: Determining Your Goals

2.) The Best Bang for Your Buzz

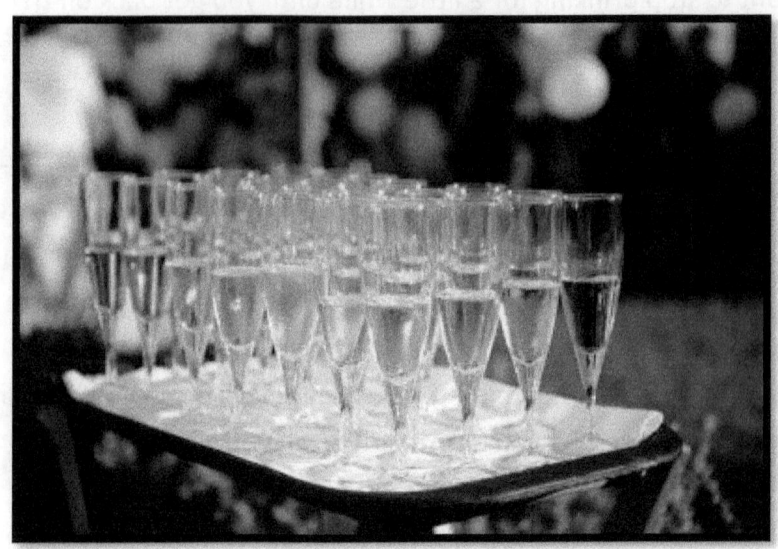

There's nothing wrong with wanting to let loose and have a little fun. For many people, that means having a drink with friends at the end of a long day or simply kicking back at home with a beer or two. If you are trying to lose weight or improve your health, however, drinking too much could interfere with your goals.

So what can you do?

The answer is simple – you just have to choose the drink that gives you the best bang for your buzz. Choosing drinks with a higher alcohol content and a low calorie count will get you where you want to be without significantly increasing your daily calorie

Chapter Two: Determining Your Goals

count. You still need to keep your goals in mind and always drink responsibly. In the next section you will find information about the calorie count of popular drinks that should be avoided if you are trying to lose weight.

1.) Calorie-Dense Drinks

If you are trying to whittle your waistline, there are certain drinks which you should avoid. You may think that distilled liquors like rum, vodka, and whiskey are a good choice because they pack a punch in terms of alcohol content. While this may be true, distilled liquors are also much more calorie-dense than wine and other drinks. Distilled liquors contain about 80 calories per ounce which is twice the calorie content as fortified wines and nearly three times the calorie content of table wines. Distilled liquors like vodka and gin also contain 8 times the calorie count of dark beers like Guinness. Who would have guessed?

<u>In order to keep your calorie count down without sacrificing your buzz, keep in mind the calorie count of certain drinks:</u>

Caloric Density of Popular Drinks		
Category	Type of Drink	Calories per Ounce
Distilled Liquor	50% ABV*	82
Distilled Liquor	40% ABV*	65

Chapter Two: Determining Your Goals

Wine	Sweet Dessert Wine	48
Wine	Port	47
Wine	White Wine	25
Wine	Red Wine	25
Beer	Sierra Nevada IPA	20
Wine	Sparkling Wine	19
Beer	Regular Beer	16
Beer	Guinness (Dark Beer)	12
Beer	Light Beer	10

*ABV = Alcohol by Volume

When considering the information listed in the table above, you also need to take into account the fact that people typically do not drink alcohol by the ounce. The serving sizes of different types of alcohol vary greatly. For example, a serving of whisky or scotch would be much smaller than a serving of wine or beer. <u>Consult the chart on the following page for a comparison of the caloric density of popular drinks by serving</u>:

Serving Sizes:

- Liquor – 1.5 oz.
- Wine – 5 oz. (4 oz. for sweet, sparkling)
- Beer – 12 oz.

Chapter Two: Determining Your Goals

Caloric Density of Popular Drinks		
Category	**Type of Drink**	**Calories per Serving**
Distilled Liquor	50% ABV*	125
Distilled Liquor	40% ABV*	98
Wine	Sweet Dessert Wine	190
Wine	Port	188
Wine	White Wine	130
Wine	Red Wine	130
Beer	Sierra Nevada IPA	240
Wine	Sparkling Wine	75
Beer	Regular Beer	155
Beer	Guinness (Dark Beer)	128
Beer	Light Beer	110

*ABV = Alcohol by Volume

When considering the information above you should also think about the fact that when you go out to drink you probably do not stop after one beverage. For most people, three drinks is the average so you can see how quickly the calories add up over the course of a night of drinking. While a glass of regular beer may only contain 155 calories or so, the number of glasses you need to get buzzed could put your calorie count well over 500. In the next section you will receive tips for finding the drinks that give you the best bang for your buzz.

2.) Low-Calorie, High Alcohol Drinks

Chapter Two: Determining Your Goals

Given the information in the previous section, you can see how certain drinks are more calorie dense than others. You also need to think about the serving size. While Sierra Nevada IPA may only contain 20 calories per ounce, a serving contains 12 ounces which puts the total calorie count for one drink at over 200. Distilled liquors, on the other hand, contain between 65 and 80 calories per ounce on average but they have a much higher alcohol content than beer and wine.

Below you will find a chart detailing the alcohol content of popular drinks to help you determine which drinks will give you the best bang for your buzz:

Alcohol Content of Popular Drinks

Category	Type of Drink	Alcohol Content (grams per calorie)
Distilled Liquor	50% ABV*	0.175
Distilled Liquor	40% ABV*	0.18
Wine	Sweet Dessert Wine	0.05
Wine	Port	0.128
Wine	White Wine	0.128
Wine	Red Wine	0.13
Beer	Sierra Nevada IPA	0.10
Wine	Sparkling Wine	0.185
Beer	Regular Beer	0.11

Chapter Two: Determining Your Goals

Beer	Guinness (Dark Beer)	0.12
Beer	Light Beer	0.13

*ABV = Alcohol by Volume

Given the information listed in the chart above, sparkling wine has the highest amount of alcohol per calorie – about 0.185 grams of alcohol per calorie. That makes it the drink that provides the best bang for your buzz. Following close behind sparkling wine are distilled liquors. The drinks next in line, port wine and white wine, sit almost 0.05 grams per calorie lower than sparkling wine. So, if you are looking for a low-calorie drink that will get you buzzed quickly, go for sparkling wine or distilled liquors.

***Note**: When drinking distilled liquors you need to factor in the calorie count of any mixer you use. To keep the calorie count down, choose diet soda or club soda.

Chapter Three: Alcohol's Effects on the Body

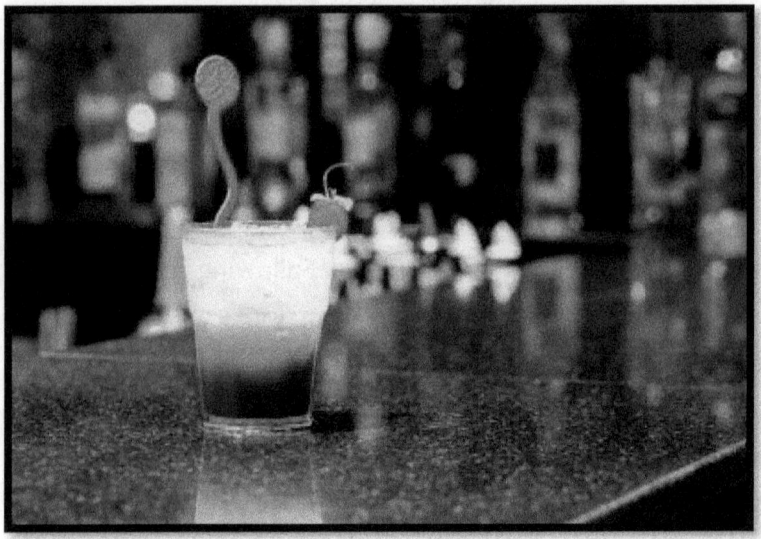

You already know that drinking alcohol can get you "buzzed" or, if you drink a little more, completely inebriated. But what else does alcohol do to your body? Drinking to excess is never a good idea but even drinking in moderation can have some significant impacts on the body such as causing dehydration, weakening the immune system, and accelerating aging. In this chapter you will learn about the various effects alcohol can have on the body both for the short-term and the long-term. Understanding the effects of alcohol will help you to make smart decisions about your drinking habits.

Chapter Three: Alcohol's Effects on the Body

1.) *Understanding the Effects of Alcohol*

Alcohol affects your body in a number of ways. Not only can it dehydrate your body by causing you to excrete (urinate) more fluids than you are taking in but it can also impair your body's natural hormone regulation. Understanding the way alcohol affects your body is very important, especially if you are trying to lose weight. In this section you will learn about how alcohol has the following effects on your body:

- Dehydration
- Accelerated aging
- Weakening the immune system
- Impairing hormone regulation
- Lack of nutrients
- Food cravings and poor eating habits
- Stimulated insulin production

Dehydrating Effects of Alcohol

One of the short-term side effects of drinking alcohol is excessive urination. This may sound strange considering the fact that beer is about 95% water. The truth of the matter is, however, that if you consume about 200 milliliters of beer (which equates to roughly 200 milliliters of water) you actually end up urinating 320 milliliters. Where does the extra come from? For one thing, your body produces about 1 milliliter of urine per kilogram of bodyweight per hour. Secondly, alcohol consumption interferes with the body's natural fluid regulation system. Alcohol induces

Chapter Three: Alcohol's Effects on the Body

the body to reduce production of anti-diuretic hormone (ADH) – as a result, your urine production increases. As you urinate more, however, your electrolyte balance remains low causing you to become dehydrated.

Alcohol and Accelerated Aging

The dehydrating effects of alcohol are closely linked to accelerated aging. As your body is forced to send the kidneys into overdrive to combat excess water levels in your body, your other organs are starved for water. Dry skin wrinkles more easily than hydrated skin and it can take on a gray pallor. Drinking alcohol can also lead to a skin condition called rosacea and puffiness in the cheeks. Other beauty-related effects of alcohol consumption include red eyes, hair loss, and dry hair.

Alcohol and the Immune System

Drinking to excess can impair the ability of the immune system to fight off disease and infections in two ways – by causing nutritional deficiency and by reducing your white blood cell count. Consumption of alcohol inhibits your body's normal ability to digest nutrients resulting from damage to the intestinal tract – it may also inhibit your liver from storing vital nutrients. A reduced number of white blood cells can reduce your body's ability to kill germs and to fight off infection – it can even lead to the development of serious conditions like cancer.

Chapter Three: Alcohol's Effects on the Body

Impaired Hormone Regulation

The endocrine system is the part of your body that produces hormones – these hormones help to stimulate growth, regulate metabolism, and influence mood. Drinking alcohol hinders the ability of your endocrine glands to secrete and regulate important hormones which can have a number of serious long-term effects. Drinking alcohol affects your body's ability to absorb nutrients which can lead to osteoporosis and it may cause other long-term problems like liver damage, ulcers, and sexual dysfunction.

Nutrients and Food Cravings

Alcohol is nearly devoid of nutrients and it can cause damage to the digestive tract which interferes with the absorption of healthy nutrients. Excessive drinking may also cause liver damage which could impair your liver's ability to store important vitamins. In addition to impacting your body's ability to absorb nutrients, drinking alcohol can also lead to food cravings. Because alcohol consists primarily of simple carbohydrates, sugar, and ethanol it often leads to food cravings which lead to overindulgence and the consumption of excess calories.

Stimulated Insulin Production

The effects of alcohol on insulin production are closely linked to the effects of alcohol on the endocrine system. Your body uses glucose for growth and for energy – that glucose comes from the

Chapter Three: Alcohol's Effects on the Body

food you eat and from the breakdown of stored glycogen in your muscles. Insulin and glucagon are the two hormones primarily responsible for the regulation of glucose levels in the blood and the function of these hormones can be impaired by alcohol consumption. Because alcohol is treated as a poison by the body, the body goes to great lengths to get rid of it and, in doing so, it may cease other important functions like regulating your blood glucose levels. Heavy drinking can lead to severe long-term effects like high blood sugar levels, liver disease, and diabetes.

Chapter Three: Alcohol's Effects on the Body

2.) Alcohol and Fat Storage – Beer Belly

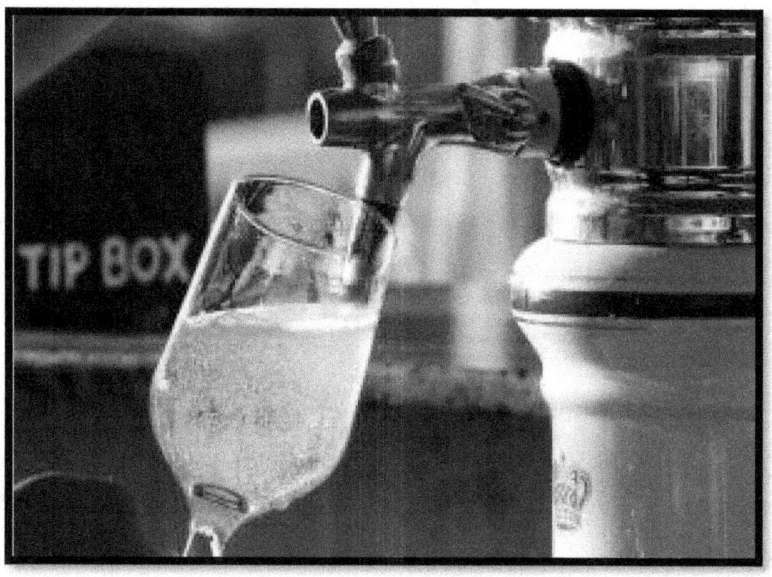

We all have that one friend who drinks on a daily basis but never seems to gain a pound. "How is that possible," you may be asking yourself. It is a combination of factors including what you drink, when you drink it, and what you eat before/while you drink. In 2010, a study was published in the *Archives of Internal Medicine* which revealed that women who had one or two alcoholic beverages per day were less likely to gain weight than those who rarely drank. The study also showed that those women who consumed alcohol daily consumed more calories daily than those who abstained from drinking.

Chapter Three: Alcohol's Effects on the Body

According to recent research, the bodies of people who drink moderately on a regular basis have adapted in such a way that they metabolize alcohol differently than the bodies of heavy drinkers or non-drinkers. The bodies of moderate regular drinkers burn the calories they drink while digesting it rather than storing those calories as fat. This is possible because the body adjusts metabolically to accommodate for the amount you drink – when you don't drink on a regular basis, your body can't make that adjustment so you end up with stored fat.

The study published in the *Archives of Internal Medicine* also showed that those who drink moderately on a regular basis are also more likely to compensate for their drinking. Women who drink regularly adjust their diet or incorporate exercise to make up for the excess calories they consume in the form of alcoholic beverages. The key is moderation – the women studied were served no more than two 1.5-ounce shots of liquor or two 4-ounce glasses of wine per day. If you drink to excess your body will only be able to compensate so much.

Chapter Three: Alcohol's Effects on the Body

a.) What Causes Beer Belly?

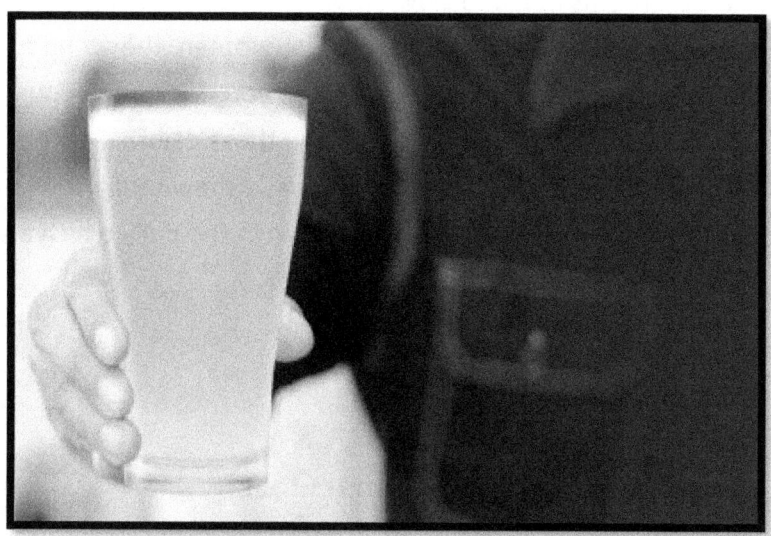

While you may be able to get away with one or two drinks a day without any negative impact on your waistline, regular overindulgence in high-carb and high-calorie beverages may lead to abdominal obesity or, and it is commonly known, beer belly. Your body reacts to alcohol in a different way than it does to food. Calories from alcohol cannot be stored for future energy in the way that food can – drinking alcohol causes your body to put your metabolism on pause. Rather than continuing to metabolize the calories from the food you just ate, your body switches over to metabolizing those alcohol calories – as a result, the calories from the food you ate gets stored as fat.

Chapter Three: Alcohol's Effects on the Body

Another factor that comes into play with "beer belly" is your age and sex. Studies have shown that once men reach the age of 35, their metabolisms begin to slow down. Extra calories are stored as fat in the abdominal area whereas, for women, they tend to be stored in the hips and backside. When you drink beer, your liver kicks into overdrive in order to burn those calories instead of burning fat like it should be. Studies have shown that drinking alcohol also decreases the rate of fat burn in the belly which also contributes to beer belly.

b.) The Dangers of Abdominal Obesity

As it has already been mentioned, beer belly is another name for abdominal obesity. Abdominal obesity occurs when you take in more calories than your body can burn – those extra calories are then stored as fat. Where that fat is stored largely depends on your age and sex. For men it is typically in the belly – for women, it is typically the hips, thighs, and buttocks. Beer belly tends to occur more in older individuals because, as you age, your metabolism slows and your daily calorie needs decrease. If you continue to eat and drink the way you did when you were young, you are likely to gain weight.

Carrying extra weight around your midsection does more than impact your physical appearance – it can have some very real consequences for your health as well. Abdominal obesity is closely associated with an increased risk for heart disease and metabolic syndrome as well as serious diseases like diabetes.

How is this risk calculated? Abdominal obesity is evaluated using several tools. The most accurate method is to take an MRI or CT scan to measure the amount of visceral fat on your body. For most people, however, a more realistic method of calculation is to take your waist-to-hip ratio. To do so, stand upright with your abdomen relaxed and measure your waist at the navel. Record this measurement then measure your hips at their widest point – this is usually in line with the bony prominences. Once you have these measurements, divide your waist measurement by your hip measurement to get your waist-to-hip ratio.

After calculating your ratio, you can determine your level of health risk. For men, a waist-to-hip ratio over 0.95 increases the risk for heart attack and stroke. For women, that number is 0.85. Another method of determining your risk is to simply take your waist circumference at the navel. Men with a waist circumference of 37 inches or less and women with a circumference below 31.5 have a low risk of heart attack and stroke. For men with a waist circumference of 37.1 to 39.9 inches and women with a circumference of 31.6 to 34.9, there is an intermediate risk. High risk is for men with a waist circumference of 40 inches or more and women with a circumference of 35 inches or more.

Chapter Three: Alcohol's Effects on the Body

c.) Gluten Sensitivity

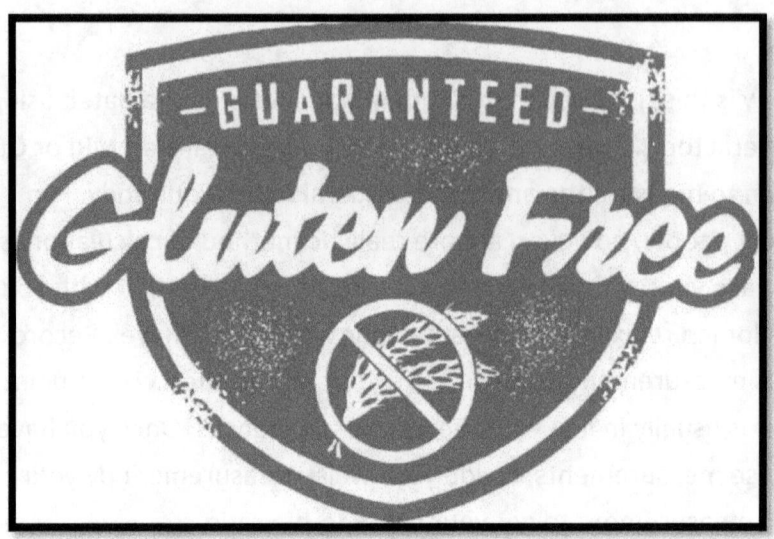

Another factor that can contribute to health problems including abdominal obesity is gluten sensitivity. Gluten is a type of protein found in certain types of grain including wheat, barley, and rye. Because these grains are often used to create beer, most beers also contain gluten. Individuals with gluten sensitivity often experience symptoms including headache, brain fog, joint pain, diarrhea, constipation, fatigue, and numbness after consuming gluten. In cases of Celiac disease, these symptoms are accompanied by the production of antibodies, autoimmune activity and damage to the lining of the intestine.

Gluten sensitivity contributes to abdominal obesity in several ways. For one thing, gluten (and wheat-based foods in general) is

Chapter Three: Alcohol's Effects on the Body

very addictive – it can cause severe food cravings which lead you to consume more food. Gluten is also very inflammatory which can lead to a number of health problems including diabetes, heart disease, and obesity. Reducing your consumption of gluten can not only provide relief from the symptoms listed earlier but it may also help you to reach your weight loss goals. If you plan to incorporate alcohol into your weight loss plan, consider switching to gluten-free varieties. You will find a number of gluten-free alcohol brands and varieties listed in the following pages.

Gluten-Free Beers

Craft breweries have begun to produce a variety of gluten-free beers and even some major brands have started to offer gluten-free varieties.

- Against the Grain
- Bards Beer
- Billabong Brewing
- EstrellaDammDaura
- Glutenberg
- Green's Gluten-Free Beer
- Hambleton Ales
- Lammsbräu
- Messagère
- New Grist
- New Planet Beer
- Omission Beer
- Ramapo Valley Brewery
- Rebellion Brewing
- RedBridge Beer
- SchitzerBräu
- Sprecher's Gluten-Free Beer
- St. Peter's
- Toleration
- TummaKukko

Chapter Three: Alcohol's Effects on the Body

Gluten-Free Hard Cider

Another great alternative to beer if you are gluten sensitive or gluten-intolerant is hard cider. The following hard cider brands are gluten-free:

- Ace Pear
- Angry Orchard
- Blue Mountain
- Blackthorn
- Bulmer's
- Crispin Cider
- Lazy Jack's
- Magner's
- Newton's Folly
- Original Sin
- Spire Mountain
- Strongbow
- Woodchuck
- Woodpecker

Most distilled liquor is gluten-free, even if it is made from wheat because the gluten protein is supposed to be removed during the distillation process. For individuals with gluten sensitivity, this is usually good enough but, if you have Celiac disease or a gluten allergy, you may still want to stay away from liquors made from gluten-containing grains. <u>Below you will find a list of popular alcohol brands that are gluten-free</u>:

Vodka

Vodka is one of those liquors that is often made from wheat. There are, however, vodkas made from potato, corn, or grapes which are safe for individuals with Celiac disease or gluten-sensitivity.

- Absolut
- Blue Ice
- Bombora

Chapter Three: Alcohol's Effects on the Body

- Chopin
- Ciroc
- Kamachatka
- Krome
- Smirnoff
- Three Olives

Tequila

When made the traditional way, tequila is produced from the agave plant so it is naturally gluten-free. Some cheaper brands, however, contain gluten so look for brands that say 100% agave on the bottle.

- 1519
- 1800
- CaboWabo
- Cazadores
- Don Julio
- El Jimador
- Herradura
- Hornitos
- Jose Cuervo
- Patron
- Suaza

Rum

- Bacardi Gold
- Bacardi Superior
- Bacardi 151
- Bacardi (flavored)
- Bundaberg
- Bayou
- Captain Morgan
- Cruzan
- Malibu
- Mount Gay
- Myer's
- Myer's Dark

Other Liquor

- Bailey's Irish Cream
- Brandy
- Campari
- Cointreau
- Fireball Cinnamon Whisky

Chapter Three: Alcohol's Effects on the Body

- Hendrick's Gin
- Hennessy Cognac
- Jack Daniels
- Jagermeister
- Jameson Irish Whisky
- Johnnie Walker Scotch
- Kahlua
- Midori
- Prosecco
- Sambuca
- Skinny Girl
- Wild Turkey Bourbon

d.) Best Beers to Drink

Even if you choose not to drink gluten-free beer, you can still make smart decisions about which beers you DO drink. The following beers are known for having a low calorie count but a comparatively high alcohol content. This means that you can achieve your desired level of inebriation without consuming too many excess calories.

Best Beers by Calorie and Alcohol Content

Type of Beer	Calorie Count	Percent Alcohol
Beck's Light	64 calories	3.8%
Milwaukee's Best Light	98 calories	4.5%
Natural Light	95 calories	4.2%
Miller Genuine Draft 64	64 calories	2.8%
Miller Lite	96 calories	4.2%

Chapter Three: Alcohol's Effects on the Body

Aspen Edge	94 calories	4.1%
Budweiser Select	99 calories	4.3%
Michelob Ultra	95 calories	4.1%
Keystone Ice	142 calories	4.1%
Corona Light	109 calories	4.5%
Milwaukee's Best Ice	144 calories	5.9%

Chapter Three: Alcohol's Effects on the Body

3.) Water and Alcohol

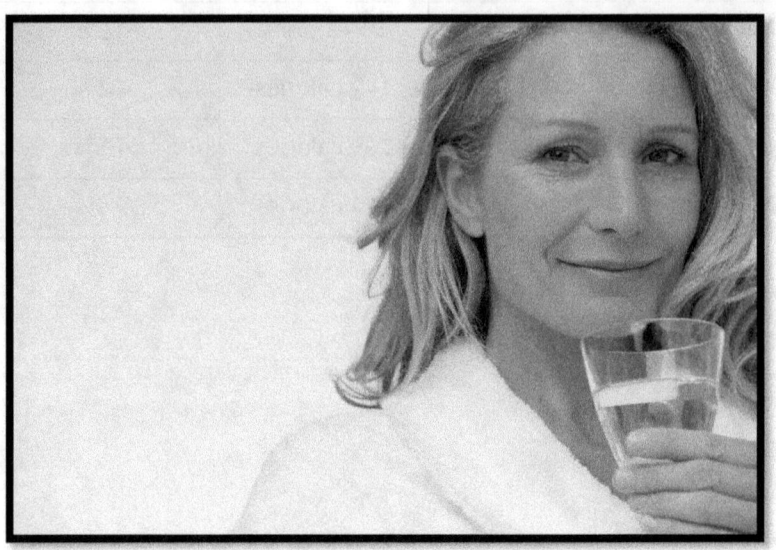

The human body is capable of surviving for weeks with no food but only 5 to 7 days without water. You become thirsty when a mere 1% of your fluid levels is lost and at 5% you begin to experience muscle cramps, decreased endurance, and fatigue. At a 10% loss of water you may become delirious and, by the time you reach a 20% loss, death is not far behind. All of this is to say that water is incredibly important for the body, not just in relation to drinking.

Chapter Three: Alcohol's Effects on the Body

a.) Water and Your Health

The male human body contains about 60% water and the female body about 50%. Your organs are the primary keepers for all this water, with your brain being one of the largest water-storing organ. Your brain is made up of about 95% water, your skin 72%, and your bones even contain about 22% water. Now you should understand just how much water your body contains, but why exactly is what so important for your health? Simply put, without water your body would not be able to function.

One of the primary functions water serves in the body is as a lubricant for various bodily processes including digestion. The water contained in your saliva carries digestive enzymes and helps to facilitate the acts of chewing and swallowing food. Water also acts as a lubricant for your cartilage and joints, helping them to move smoothly. Water also plays an important role in regulating your body temperature. The body controls over-heating by sweating - that is releasing perspiration from sweat glands in the skin. In the cold, your body moves blood away from the surface to conserve body heat.

Another way water works in the body is to help flush toxins and waste out of your system through both urination and perspiration. When you are properly hydrated, your bowel movements also help to ensure that wastes are removed quickly and efficiently from the body. Your blood contains about 92%

Chapter Three: Alcohol's Effects on the Body

water and it is responsible for carrying oxygen and valuable nutrients throughout the body. Many nutrients are water-soluble which means that they can be dissolved in water so they can pass through the capillaries in the walls of the intestine where they are absorbed and distributed throughout the body.

Drinking enough water on a daily basis is incredibly important. If you drink eight glasses of water per day, your risk for colon cancer could be reduced by 45% and your risk for bladder cancer by 50% - drinking plenty of water may also reduce your risk for breast cancer. Staying hydrated throughout the day will also help you to avoid the symptoms of dehydration which may include headache, fatigue, blurred vision and joint pain.

b.) Staying Hydrated While Drinking

When you consume an alcoholic beverage, your body expels up to four times the volume of that beverage through urine which can quickly lead to dehydration if you are not careful. The key to avoiding a nasty hangover is to follow each alcoholic beverage with an 8-ounce glass of water. Another tip for staying hydrated is to order your drinks "on the rocks," or over ice. As the ice in your drink melts it becomes more diluted. Drinking more slowly can also help to prevent dehydration because your body can absorb alcohol more quickly than it can metabolize it. If you sip your drink slowly your body will be able to process it much more effectively than if you chug it all at once.

According to research conducted at the University of Manchester, pairing alcohol with carbonated mixers can increase the rate of alcohol absorption into your blood. As an alternative, use mixers like fruit juice or water. If you do use carbonated mixers, try to alternate between alcoholic and non-alcoholic beverages. If you are at a party and are worried about keeping up appearances, you can also order a drink that looks alcoholic – a glass of coke without the rum or some ginger ale in a wine glass. No one will be the wiser.

c.) Rehydrating the Day After

Depending how much water you drank the night before, you may wake up after a night of drinking with a nasty hangover. So what do you do to rehydrate your body? Drinking a few glasses of water may not be enough – you also need to replenish your electrolyte stores. Drinking a sports drink is one way to get some extra electrolytes but you can also just add a pinch of sea salt to a glass of water as well. If you're feeling a bit queasy, try a glass of ginger ale to soothe your upset stomach while also helping to restore your fluid balance.

Chapter Three: Alcohol's Effects on the Body

4.) Sleep and Alcohol

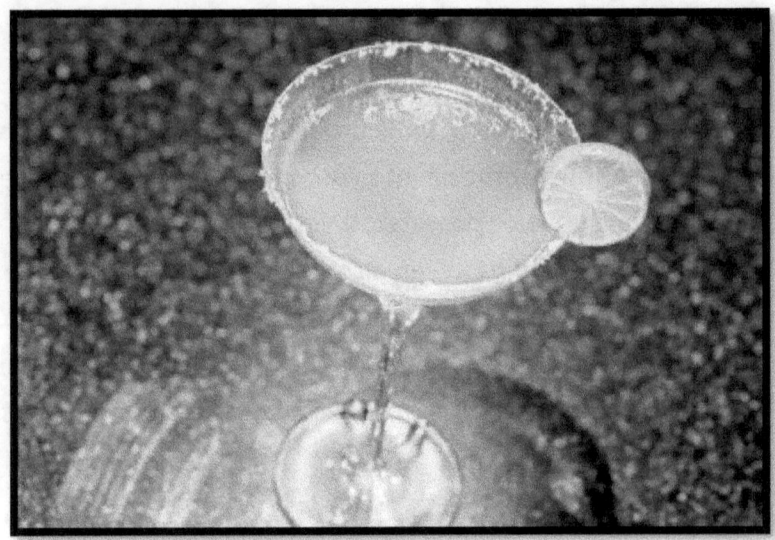

Sleep is incredibly important for your health, though many people do not get the sleep they need. According to the National Sleep Foundation your sleep needs are impacted by your health and lifestyle – your needs for sleep may vary significantly from someone else's. Some people find that they are alert and productive after seven hours of sleep while some people need nine hours just to feel functional in the morning. One thing is universal across the board, however – consuming alcohol has a significant impact on the quality of your sleep.

When you become intoxicated, the alcohol inhibits your body's natural sleep cycle by disrupting both the sleep sequence and the

Chapter Three: Alcohol's Effects on the Body

duration of your sleep. This also affects your brain's ability to retain information because your memories become solidified while you are sleeping. After a night of drinking, your REM stage of sleep is going to be compromised – this means that you will not be getting the same quality of deep sleep that you normally would, even though you may appear to be sleeping deeply.

When you wake up after a night of drinking, you are likely to feel tired, perhaps for the whole of the next day. Heavy drinking has the potential to affect your sleep as well as other brain and body activities for up to three days. If you drink for two consecutive nights, it could affect your brain and body for up to 5 days. Even if you only have a couple drinks, you may experience a shortened attention span for up to 48 hours and you may still have a raised blood alcohol level of up to 0.03 long after you stop feeling the effects of the alcohol.

Chapter Three: Alcohol's Effects on the Body

5.) Short and Long-Term Effects

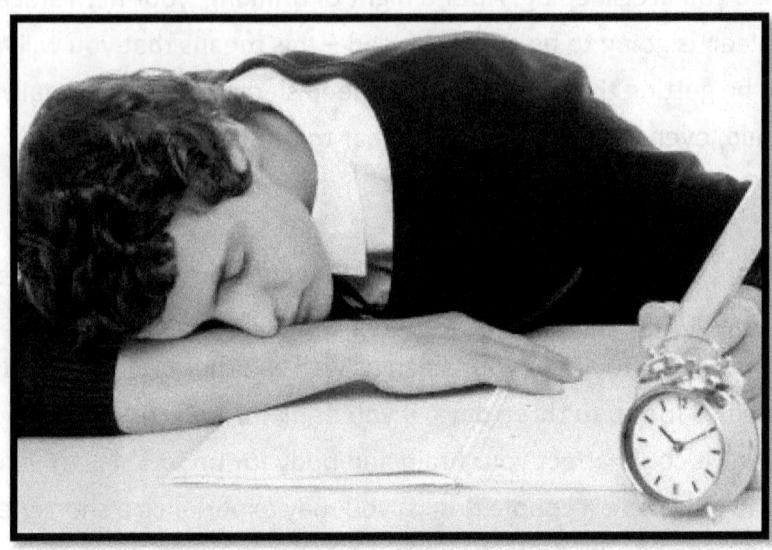

For many people, the desired benefit of drinking is to become less inhibited and to relieve stress or anxiety. There are, however, a number of other effects which you may not be counting on. Most of the effects alcohol has on the body impact the brain – when you are intoxicated, alcohol impairs the ability of your central nervous system to analyze sensory information. This is why when you are drunk you may experience blurred vision, slurred speech, decreased coordination, and dulling of pain sensations. As you continue drinking, you may experience more profound effects such as a loss of balance, loss of the ability to judge height or distance, and dizziness.

Chapter Three: Alcohol's Effects on the Body

Only about 10% of the alcohol you drink is excreted through urine or breathing – that leaves your liver to deal with the remaining 90%. The liver is capable of metabolizing alcohol at the rate of one drink per hour. This is why you could still fail a breathalyzer test the morning after heavily drinking – it also explains why drinking copious amounts of alcohol in a short period of time can be fatal. If, after a night of drinking, you wake up and continue drinking then your blood alcohol level could be much higher than you think it is.

When you drink alcohol your body responds to the rapid influx of glucose by producing higher quantities of insulin. Once this happens, your body keeps working to remove the excess glucose from your blood stream. At a certain point, your blood glucose level may become too low which could cause you to feel shaky, dizzy, and tired – you may also experience blurred vision or heavy sweating. The best way to counteract the effects of low blood glucose levels is to give your body a carbohydrate boost – this is why you often feel hungry after drinking. Your body craves carbs to make up for lost glucose and a lack of energy.

Drinking alcohol can affect more than just your judgment and your sleep – it can also have an effect on your muscles and your overall nutrition. Consuming alcohol after a workout can result in reduced protein synthesis which might impede muscle growth. Alcohol also deprives your body of human growth hormone (HGH), a hormone that is responsible for the process of building and repairing muscle. Another factor that impacts your gains from a workout is your recovery speed – drinking alcohol deprives your body of water and slows its natural healing ability.

Negative health effects related to alcohol can occur over a relatively short period of time. Depending on the amount and frequency of your drinking, addiction can occur in as little as 18 months. Genetic factors or a history of addiction could increase your risk and speed up the process. It is also worth noting that women can develop health problems related to alcohol over a shorter period of time than men. <u>Some of the long-term health problems related to alcohol include the following:</u>

- **Heart Disease** – The moderate consumption of red wine may provide health benefits for the heart, but long-term heavy drinking could increase your risk for heart disease and high blood pressure.

- **Liver Disease** – Heavy drinking can lead to inflammation of the liver or alcoholic hepatitis – if you continue drinking with this condition you could die.

- **Pancreatitis** – Long-term drinking can lead to inflammation of the pancreas, or pancreatitis.

- **Cancer** – Heavy drinking over a long period of time can increase your risk for developing certain cancers, especially mouth, throat, and esophageal cancers.

Chapter Three: Alcohol's Effects on the Body

Chapter Four: Factors that Effect Intoxication

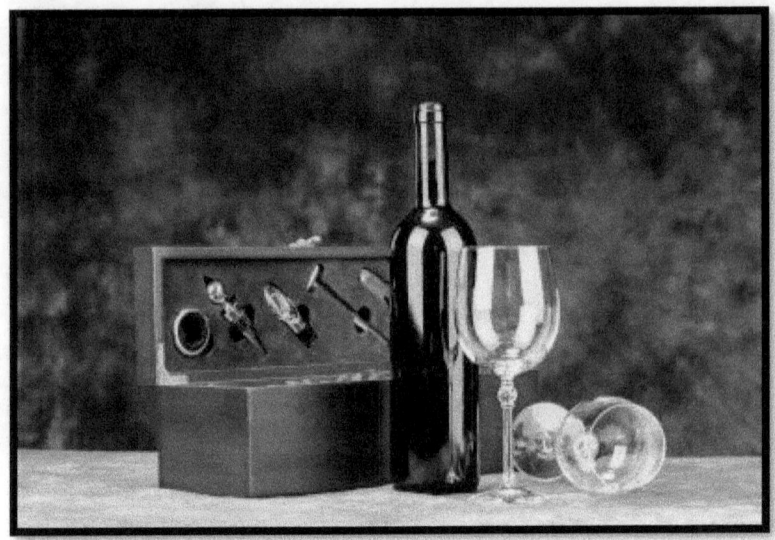

What is the difference between a person who gets sloppy after two drinks and someone who can hold their liquor for a full night of drinking? The obvious differences may be many but there may be some surprising factors that affect intoxication as well. For one thing, men and women absorb alcohol differently. Other factors such as mood, body type, even the food you eat before you drink can affect the rate of absorption and your level of intoxication. In this chapter you will learn how various factors affect your body's absorption of alcohol and what that means for your buzz.

Chapter Four: Factors that Effect Intoxication

1.) Alcohol and Food

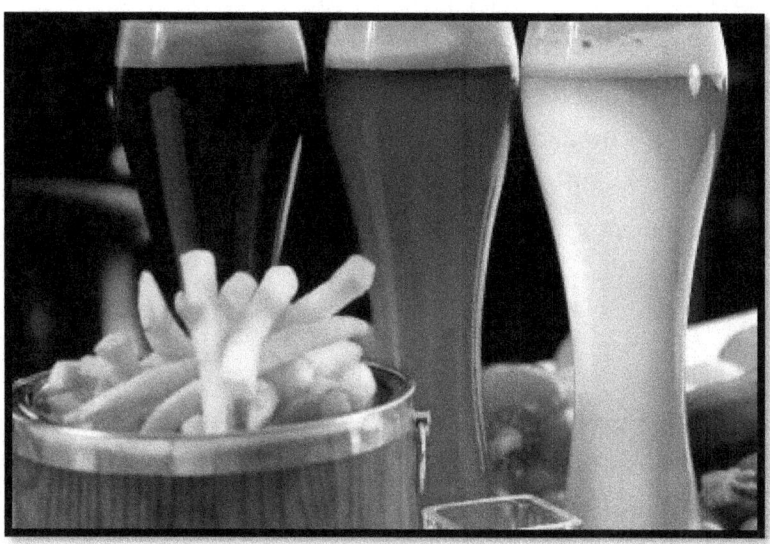

As you learned in the last chapter, your liver is only capable of digesting about one standard drink per hour. Drinking at this rate will help to keep your liver from becoming overloaded and it also helps you to achieve the desired level of buzz while maintaining a safe blood alcohol level. The food you eat and when you eat it also has an effect on your body's absorption of alcohol. For example, if you do not eat before drinking you will likely hit a peak Blood Alcohol Concentration (BAC) after about one half to two hours of drinking. If you eat before drinking, on the other hand, you'll reach your peak BAC sometime between one and six hours of drinking.

Chapter Four: Factors that Effect Intoxication

Based on this information, you can see how having a snack before you drink is a good idea. But what should you eat? Many kinds of alcohol, particularly mixed drinks, are loaded with carbohydrates which send your blood sugar skyrocketing and then crashing a few hours later. To combat this sequence you should have a meal or snack before drinking that provides fiber, protein, and healthy fat. Something like a cup of Greek yogurt with strawberries, or an apple with peanut butter should do the trick – even a protein shake if that's what you prefer.

Having some food in your stomach before you begin drinking will slow your absorption rate and it will keep you from making poor food decisions later. When you are already intoxicated and hungry, you might not see the harm in ordering a greasy hamburger loaded up with bacon even after you've eaten a full day's worth of calories. If you know you will be eating at the bar, check the menu ahead of time and decide what you are going to order. Even something like a vegetable platter with hummus can be beneficial – celery and other vegetables will also help to keep you hydrated without having to down a giant glass of water after every alcoholic drink.

Chapter Four: Factors that Effect Intoxication

2.) Body Weight and Type

Gender is a significant factor when it comes to the absorption of alcohol. For example, a male and female of the same weight might have very different BACs after consuming the same amount of alcohol in the same amount of time. A man weighing 140 pounds consumes two drinks in an hour and has a BAC of 0.038 while a female weighing 140 pounds drinks the same amount in the same hour and has a BAC of 0.048. Why does this happen?

The human stomach contains an enzyme called dehydrogenase which helps to break down alcohol. Women have less of this enzyme and thus a lesser ability to break down alcohol – as a result, a women will have a higher BAC than a man after drinking the same amount of alcohol. Women also tend to have higher body fat percentages and lower water content then men which can affect the absorption rate. This is why people with small body types and less body fat absorb alcohol at a faster rate than larger people with more body fat.

Chapter Four: Factors that Effect Intoxication

3.) Rate of Consumption/ Strength of Drink

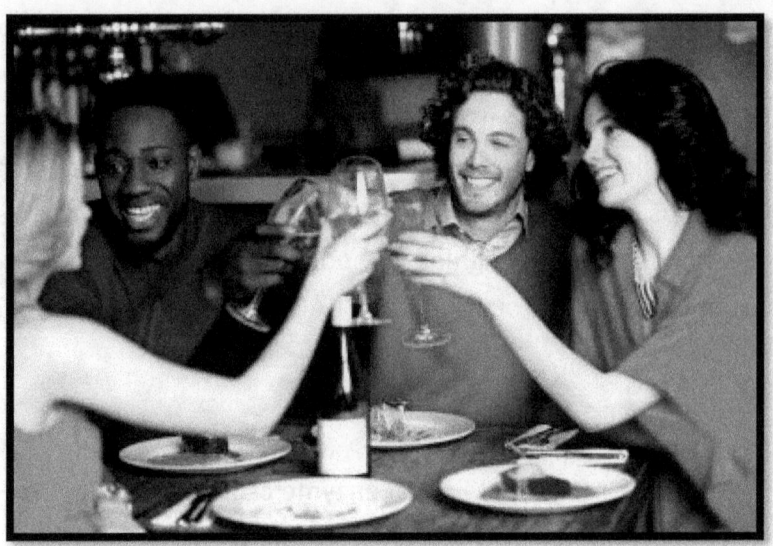

It should come as no surprise that the faster you drink, the more quickly your BAC will rise. The strength of the drink also impacts the rate of absorption – stronger drinks will increase your BAC more quickly than weak drinks. Drinks with a higher alcohol concentration irritate the mucus membranes of your digestive tract which may decrease the rate of absorption. Refer back to the information in Chapter Two to determine the alcohol content of popular drinks.

Not only do different drinks have different rates of absorption, but certain drinks can affect your appetite more than others. Having a healthy snack while drinking is a great idea to slow your

Chapter Four: Factors that Effect Intoxication

absorption rate and to keep your BAC under control, but some cocktails may cause cravings for carbs and sugar that could become problematic if you're trying to lose weight. Sweet drinks and fancy cocktails tend to be loaded with sugar which makes them not only high in calories but dangerous in terms of causing food cravings.

Chapter Four: Factors that Effect Intoxication

4.) Other Factors

Some other factors which might affect your absorption rate for alcohol include your mood, your functional tolerance level, and any medications you may be taking. Drinking alcohol has a significant impact on your mood and it can cause any feelings you had prior to drinking to become exaggerated. At a BAC between 0.02 and 0.05, you may experience a slight improvement in mood. Once you reach a BAC of 0.07, however, your mood is likely to deteriorate. If you are feeling stressed, depressed, or anxious, it could affect the way the enzymes in your stomach break down the alcohol which could impact your rate of absorption and your BAC.

Over time and with frequent drinking, your body's reaction to the effects of alcohol may decrease – this is referred to as functional tolerance. For example, if you have a high functional tolerance you may be able to drink more before you feel or exhibit the effects of alcohol than a person who has a low functional tolerance – you may hear this referred to using the term "lightweight". Even if you have a high functional tolerance, that doesn't mean anything for your BAC – it could still be high even if you aren't feeling the effects of alcohol. If you develop a functional tolerance upwards of 50% - that is, requiring twice the amount of alcohol to feel any effects – it could be a sign of a growing alcohol problem or addiction.

Chapter Four: Factors that Effect Intoxication

Another factor influencing your rate of alcohol absorption is the medications you are taking. Alcohol is technically a drug, a mind-altering substance, so it should be treated the same way as you would treat a prescription. You wouldn't mix two prescriptions without knowing what effect they are going to have, would you? In the same way you shouldn't mix alcohol with medications without first consulting your doctor to make sure it is safe.

Some medications, like anti-depressants, should never be mixed with alcohol. It is also important to note that while having a drink or two while taking some medications might be okay, drinking to excess could be incredibly dangerous. Not only can medications change the way your body reacts to alcohol, but alcohol can change the way your body reacts to your medications as well. In some cases the effects of the medication may be lessened by alcohol but in other cases they could be increased. Certain types of pain killers and cold medicines tend to multiply the effects of alcohol as much as ten times the normal amount!

Just as you would be careful with drinking while taking any medication, you should also be careful about drinking while you are sick or fatigued. When you are sick, there is also a significant risk that you are dehydrated and this could cause your BAC to climb quickly. If you are fatigued, alcohol could intensify those feelings and cause you to quickly develop a high BAC.

Chapter Five: Making a Plan for Drinking

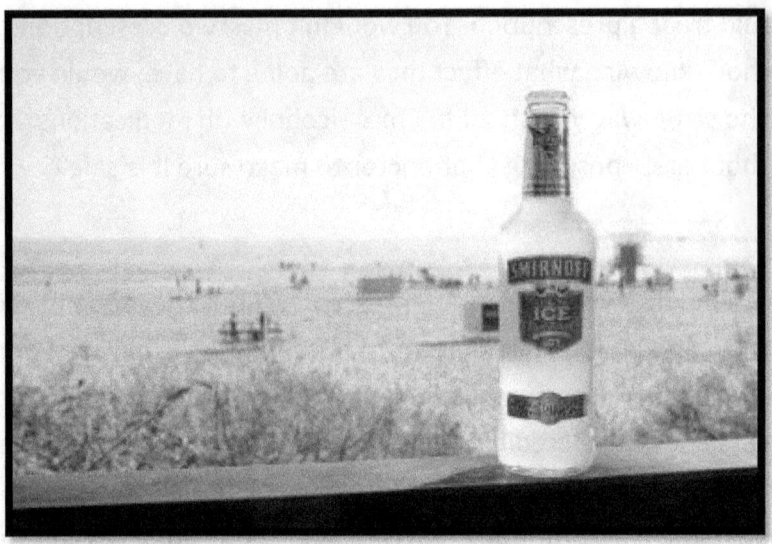

There's no harm in enjoying the occasional alcoholic beverage – we all do it! If you are striving to lose weight or to improve your health, however, you may be facing an extra challenge – how to pair your drinking with your health and fitness goals. The solution is to drink smart. Plan out the days or nights when you will be drinking and learn what to eat and drink before, during, and after your drinking as well. In this chapter you will receive tips for making a plan for drinking that won't hamper you from achieving your goals.

Chapter Five: Making a Plan for Drinking

1.) Before You Drink

The key to sticking to a healthy eating plan while still enjoying the occasional drink is to know when you are going to be drinking. Below you will find a few simple tips for staying on track when planning your next night of drinking:

1. **Never drink on an empty stomach** – drinking on an empty stomach will not only increase your rate of absorption but it can also be damaging to the lining of your intestinal tract. Once your digestive tract is damaged, it could impair your body's ability to properly absorb nutrients which could result in a variety of health problems including leaky gut syndrome.

2. **Drink some water first** – before drinking you should make sure that you are properly hydrated. It is also recommended that you alternate between alcoholic and non-alcoholic drinks during the night so you stay hydrated as you drink. It also never hurts to drink a glass of water before you go to bed – this can help to stave off a hangover.

3. **Be mindful of your mixers** – if you are trying to lose weight you may want to steer clear of sugary and high-calorie mixers like fruit juice, sour mix, and soda. Add a few ice cubes to your drink to dilute it and make it last longer or go

Chapter Five: Making a Plan for Drinking

with a low-calorie mixer like club soda.

4. **Drink responsibly** – binge drinking is never a good idea because it can be very damaging to your health. If you are going to drink, limit yourself to one or two drinks – know your own limits and do not push them.

5. **Sip your drinks slowly** – the faster you drink, the more quickly you will become intoxicated. While this may seem like a good idea after a particularly stressful day, it could result in some serious negative side effects. Your liver can only digest one drink per hour, so don't push it!

Chapter Five: Making a Plan for Drinking

2.) Before You Drink

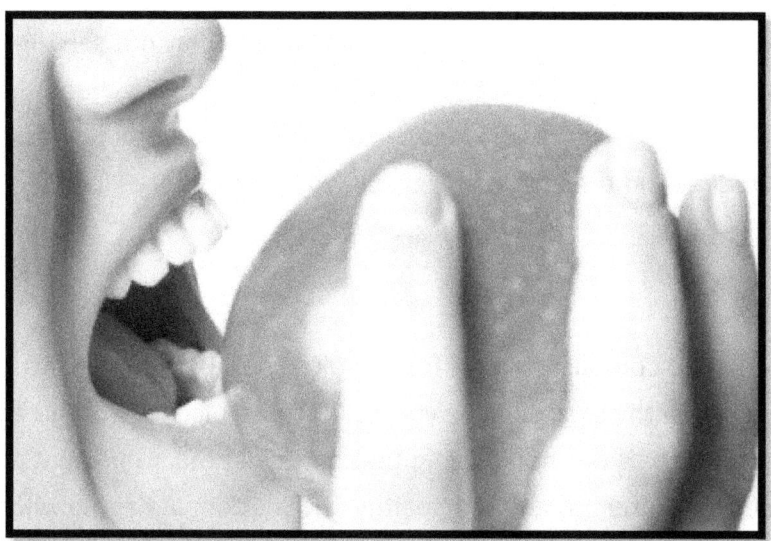

Before you go out drinking you should follow a few simple rules. First, make sure you've had plenty of water to drink during the day so you are not dehydrated – being dehydrated will increase the effects of alcohol on your body and it could cause your blood alcohol concentration to rise more quickly than you would like. Second, have a snack before you go! Many people with goals of weight loss try to restrict their eating during the day in order to "save up" calories for drinking later. This tactic tends to fail in a number of ways.

In restricting your eating before drinking you will experience a faster rate of absorption which means that you will experience

Chapter Five: Making a Plan for Drinking

the effects of alcohol more quickly. Why does this matter? Because when you become intoxicated you may lose your inhibitions, especially when it comes to eating. While the sober you might opt for a salad, the intoxicated you may not see the harm in ordering a basket of French fries drenched in cheese and chili. Drinking sugary cocktails can also cause your blood sugar to skyrocket and then to crash, leaving you craving carbs in any shape or form.

The key to combatting poor food choices during drinking is to have a healthy snack before you go. Because alcoholic drinks are high in carbs, you should avoid that particular macronutrient and focus on protein, fiber, and healthy fat. Snack on an apple with peanut butter, some beef jerky, maybe a few slices of avocado. Snacks like these will take longer for your body to break down and absorb than carb-loaded snacks which will also slow your rate of absorption for alcohol.

Chapter Five: Making a Plan for Drinking

3.) The Day After

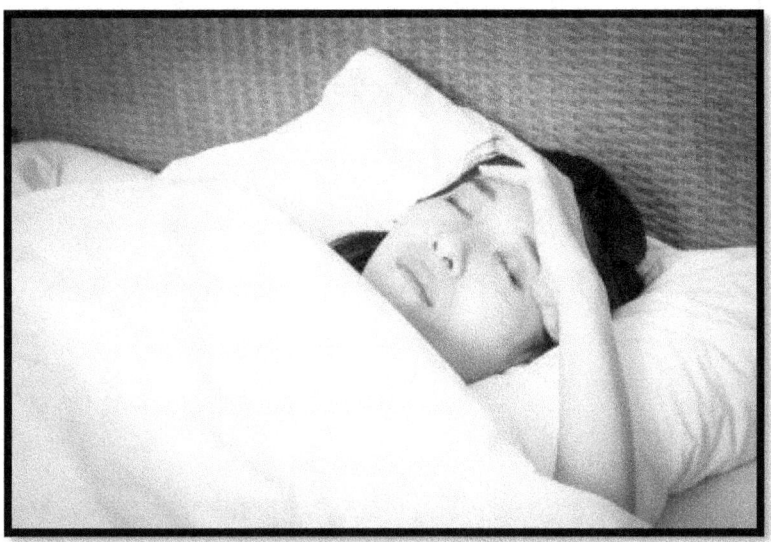

The day after a night of drinking it is important to rehydrate your body and to fuel up with some healthy nutrients. You also need to replenish your electrolyte stores to help fight off that feeling of fatigue. Try drinking a large 16-ounce glass of water with the juice of one lemon and a pinch of sea salt added. Not only will this help to rehydrate your body but it will also support two of your most important detoxification organs – your liver and your kidneys. You might also want to try some fresh juice or a green smoothie for a quick boost of nutrition.

In addition to rehydrating your body and fueling up with nutrients, you might also want to consider throwing in a little bit

Chapter Five: Making a Plan for Drinking

of exercise. A quick thirty minutes of cardio in the morning will help to get your blood flowing and it will help you to shake off that foggy feeling you sometimes have after a night of drinking. A little bit of exercise will also help to boost your metabolism which can only help in terms of your weight loss goals.

Chapter Five: Making a Plan for Drinking

a.) Day-After Juice and Smoothie Recipes

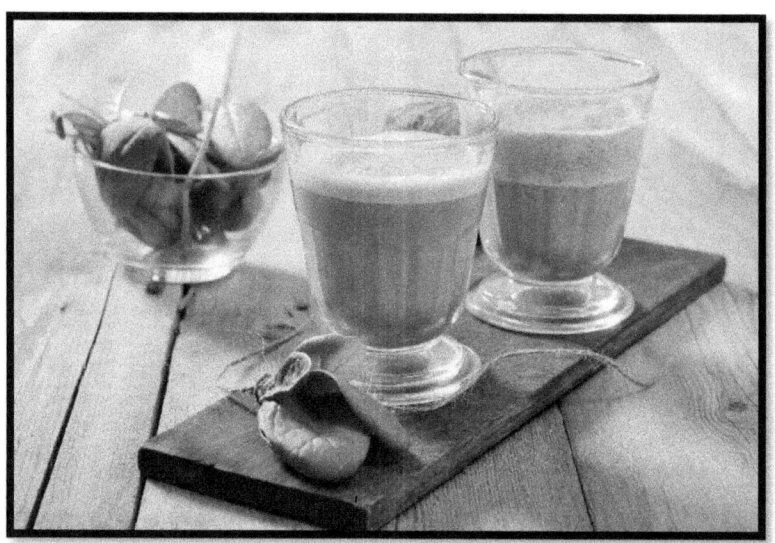

Recipes Included in this Section:

Ginger, Carrot Beet Juice

Protein-Packed Spinach Smoothie

Lemon Dandelion Green Juice

Detoxifying Coconut Smoothie

Savory Tomato Cucumber Juice

Chocolate Almond Banana Smoothie

Celery Apple Juice with Lemon

Blueberry Chia Seed Smoothie

Ginger, Carrot, Beet Juice

Servings: 1 to 2

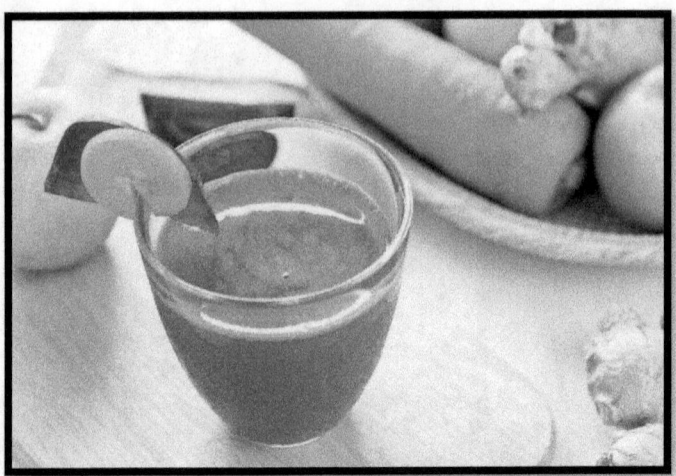

Ingredients:

- 3 large carrots, peeled
- 2 medium beets, scrubbed well
- 1 large Granny Smith apple, cored
- 1 inch fresh ginger, peeled

Instructions:

1. Wash all ingredients well and chop to size to fit the juicer.
2. Place a large glass or pitcher beneath the spout of your pitcher.
3. Feed the ingredients through the juicer in the order listed.
4. Stir your juice well then divide between two glasses (if desired) and enjoy immediately.

Chapter Five: Making a Plan for Drinking

Protein-Packed Spinach Smoothie

Servings: 1 to 2

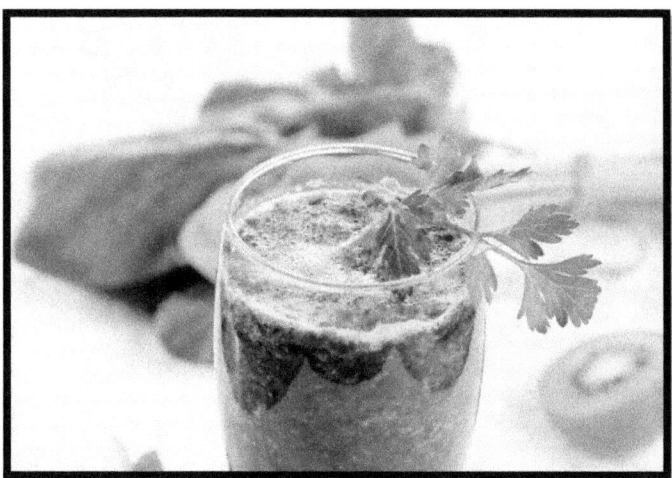

Ingredients:

- 2 cups fresh baby spinach
- 1 fresh kiwi fruit, peeled and sliced
- 1 cup fat-free milk
- ½ cup non-fat Greek yogurt
- 1 scoop protein powder
- 1 tablespoon honey

Instructions:

1. Combine all of the ingredients in a high-speed blender.
2. Blend on high speed for 30 to 60 seconds until smooth and well combined.
3. Divide between two glasses and enjoy immediately.

Chapter Five: Making a Plan for Drinking

Lemon Dandelion Green Juice

Servings: 1 to 2

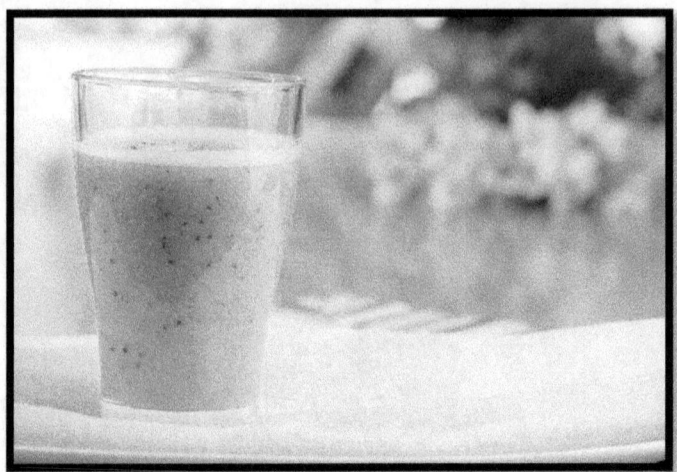

Ingredients:

- 1 bunch fresh dandelion greens
- 2 ripe kiwi fruit, peeled
- 2 medium stalks celery
- 1 ripe lemon, halved
- ½ seedless cucumber, peeled

Instructions:

1. Wash all ingredients well and chop to size to fit the juicer.
2. Place a large glass or pitcher beneath the spout of your pitcher.
3. Feed the ingredients through the juicer in the order listed.
4. Stir your juice well then divide between two glasses (if desired) and enjoy immediately.

Chapter Five: Making a Plan for Drinking

Detoxifying Coconut Smoothie

Servings: 1 to 2

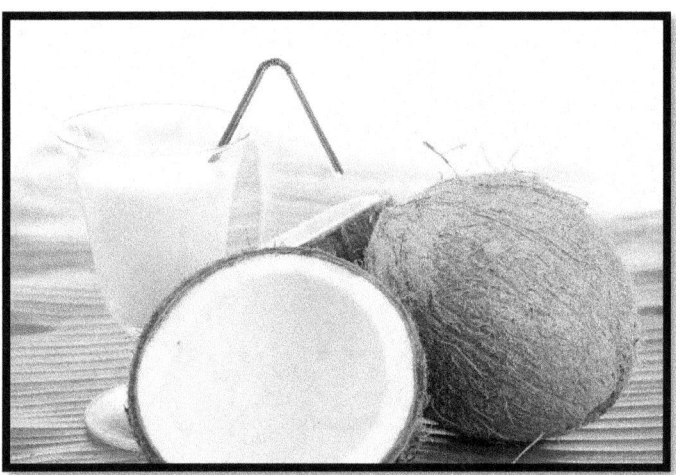

Ingredients:

- 2 cups fresh baby spinach
- 1 large frozen banana, peeled and sliced
- 1 cup unsweetened coconut milk
- ½ cup ice cubes
- ¼ cup unsweetened shredded coconut
- 1 teaspoon honey

Instructions:

1. Combine all of the ingredients in a high-speed blender.
2. Blend on high speed for 30 to 60 seconds until smooth and well combined.
3. Divide between two glasses and enjoy immediately.

Chapter Five: Making a Plan for Drinking

Savory Tomato Cucumber Juice

Servings: 1 to 2

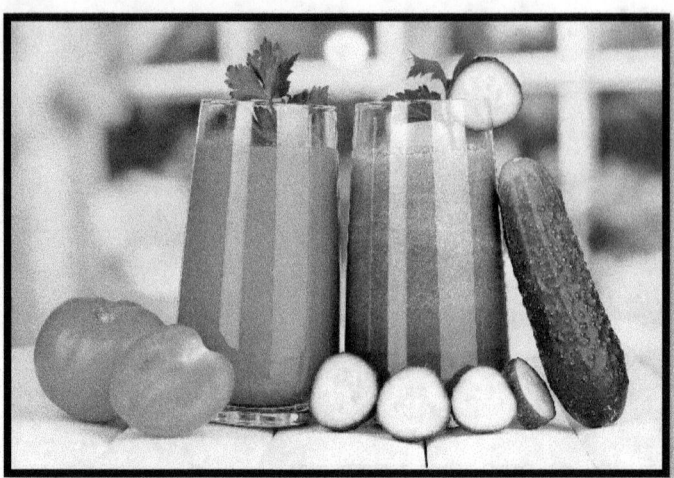

Ingredients:

- 2 medium Roma tomatoes, cored
- 1 large seedless cucumber, peeled
- 1 small carrot, chopped
- 1 clove garlic, peeled
- 2 tablespoons fresh cilantro

Instructions:

1. Wash all ingredients well and chop to size to fit the juicer.
2. Place a large glass or pitcher beneath the spout of your pitcher.
3. Feed the ingredients through the juicer in the order listed.
4. Stir your juice well then divide between two glasses (if desired) and enjoy immediately.

Chapter Five: Making a Plan for Drinking

Chocolate Almond Banana Smoothie

Servings: 1 to 2

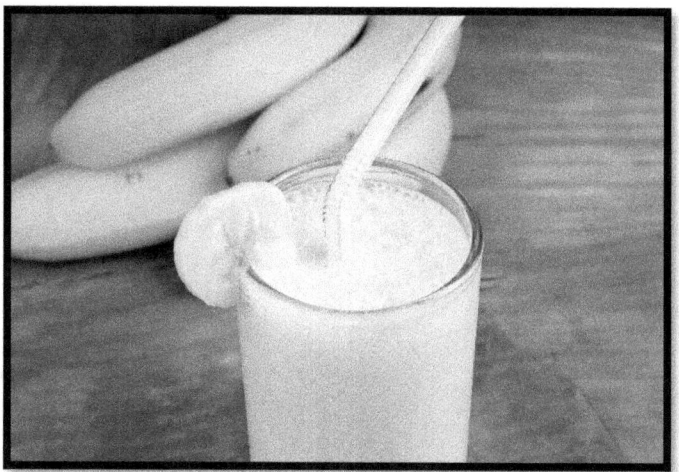

Ingredients:

- 2 medium frozen bananas, peeled and sliced
- 1 cup fat-free milk
- ¼ cup non-fat Greek yogurt
- 2 tablespoons almond butter
- 1 tablespoon unsweetened cocoa powder

Instructions:

1. Combine all of the ingredients in a high-speed blender.
2. Blend on high speed for 30 to 60 seconds until smooth and well combined.
3. Divide between two glasses and enjoy immediately.

Celery Apple Juice with Lime

Servings: 1 to 2

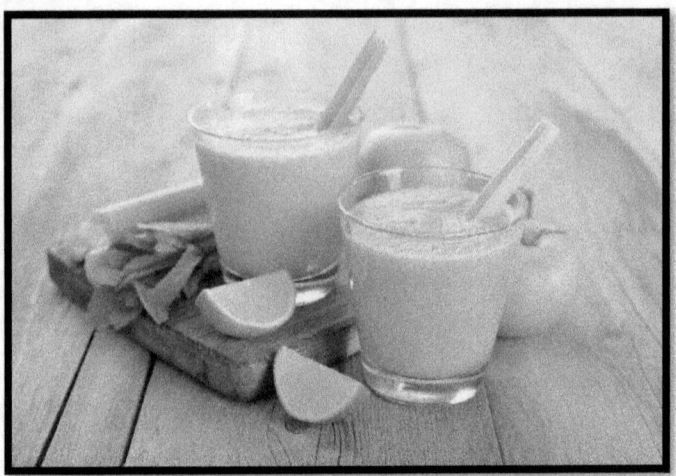

Ingredients:

- 4 large stalks celery
- 1 large Granny Smith apple, cored
- 1 cup dandelion greens
- ½ lime, peel removed

Instructions:

1. Wash all ingredients well and chop to size to fit the juicer.
2. Place a large glass or pitcher beneath the spout of your pitcher.
3. Feed the ingredients through the juicer in the order listed.
4. Stir your juice well then divide between two glasses (if desired) and enjoy immediately.

Chapter Five: Making a Plan for Drinking

Blueberry Chia Seed Smoothie

Servings: 1 to 2

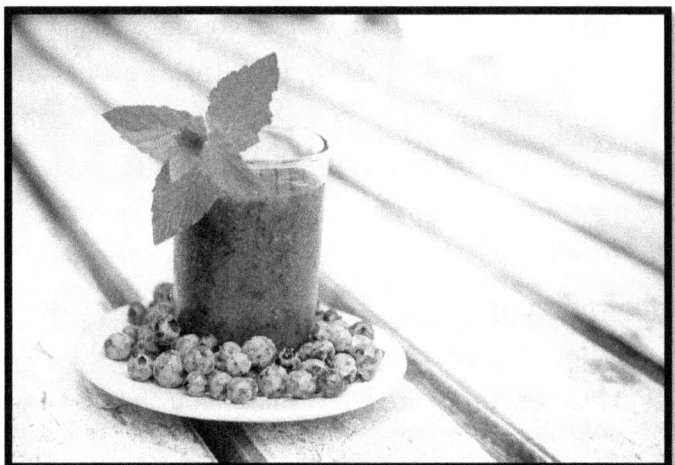

Ingredients:

- 2 cups frozen blueberries
- 1 small frozen banana, peeled and sliced
- 1 cup fat-free milk
- ½ cup non-fat Greek yogurt, plain
- 1 tablespoon chia seeds

Instructions:

1. Combine all of the ingredients in a high-speed blender.
2. Blend on high speed for 30 to 60 seconds until smooth and well combined.
3. Divide between two glasses and enjoy immediately.

Chapter Five: Making a Plan for Drinking

4.) Taking a Break

Every once in a while you might want to consider taking a break from alcohol, and not just for a few days. Taking a week or a month off from drinking could have some significant health benefits for your body. There are many reasons for taking a break from alcohol. Perhaps it is having a negative impact on your weight loss goals, maybe your friends are becoming concerned with your level of drinking, or maybe you just want to take a break for your own personal reasons. Whatever your motivation may be, there are a few things you should know.

Each time you take a drink, you start to build up a tolerance for alcohol – think back to the previous chapter and the section about functional tolerance. The age at which you begin drinking, your family history, and the frequency with which you drink all have an impact on your tolerance. If your tolerance becomes too high, it could skew your understanding of how much is "too much" – even if you cut back on your drinking you might still be consuming more than a normal or healthy amount. A high tolerance might also result in you making risky decisions or poor judgment calls because you feel "normal" despite having a high BAC level.

Before you take a break from alcohol, take the time to seriously think about your reasons. If you are reacting to concern from friends or family, think about the ways your drinking might be

Chapter Five: Making a Plan for Drinking

affecting them and use that information as motivation to stay strong during your break. If your drinking is having an impact on your work or day-to-day life, make note of the specific ways it is impeding you and make note of how you'd like to see those areas of your life improve during your break. Perhaps your drinking is putting a strain on your finances or maybe you just want the peace of mind in knowing that you can stop if you want to. Whatever your motivation may be, take the time to identify and understand it before you start your break.

When taking a break from alcohol you need to decide ahead of time exactly how long the break will be. Do not let yourself cut the break short because things get hard – stay true to yourself and to your motivations for taking the break in the first place. Depending on your level and frequency of drinking before the break you may experience some symptoms of withdrawal such as nausea, perspiration, rapid pulse, hallucinations, irritability, depression, aggression, anxiety, and insomnia. If you have a serious drinking problem, you should consult your doctor for help with the withdrawal symptoms.

Chapter Six: Highest and Lowest Calorie Drinks

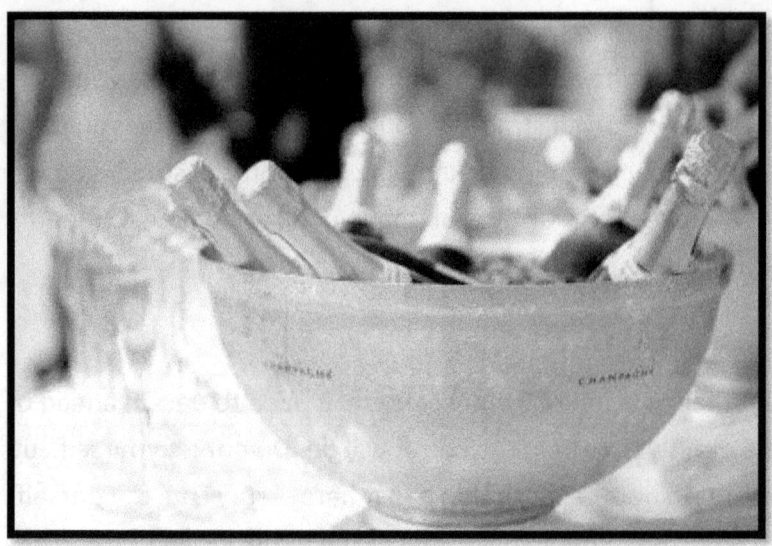

When you are trying to lose weight, it is important to know the calorie content of the food you consume and the beverages you drink. You may not realize that the cocktail you are idly sipping on at the bar on Friday night contains nearly 300 calories or that this same beverage could cause food cravings which will have you diving to the bottom of the bowl of salty snack mix the bartender sets before you. In this chapter you will receive a list of some of the most popular high-calorie and low-calorie cocktails so you have an idea what to order when you decide to go out for a drink or two.

Chapter Six: Highest and Lowest Calorie Drinks

1.) Highest Calorie Cocktails

<u>Below you will find a list of some of the highest-calorie cocktails(over 200 calories) that you should avoid if you are trying to lose weight</u>:

- Long Island Iced Tea – 500 to 700 calories
- Frozen Margarita – 500 to 700 calories
- Frozen Daiquiri – 500 to 600 calories
- Pina Colada – 400 to 600 calories
- Chocolate Martini – 450 calories
- White Russian – 400 calories
- Mai Tai – 300 calories
- Hot Buttered Rum – 300 calories
- Wine Coolers – 250 calories
- Gin and Tonic –250 calories
- Cosmopolitan – 200 calories
- Vodka and Tonic – 200 calories

Chapter Six: Highest and Lowest Calorie Drinks

2.) *Lowest Calorie Cocktails*

<u>Below you will find a list of some of the lowest calorie drinks cocktails (under 200 calories) that will help to prevent you from going over your calorie goal on days you drink:</u>

- Screwdriver (8 oz.) – 190 calories
- Rum and Coke (8 oz.) – 185 calories
- Vodka Martini – 160 calories
- Regular Beer (12 oz.) – 150 to 200 calories
- Green Apple Martini – 150 calories
- Spiced Cider with Rum (8 oz.) – 150 calories
- Port Wine (3 oz.) – 130 calories
- Bloody Mary (5 oz.) – 120 calories
- Red Wine (5 oz.) – 120 calories
- White Wine (5 oz.) – 120 calories
- Light Beer (12 oz.) – 100 to 140 calories
- Wine Spritzer (5 oz.) – 100 calories
- Rum and Diet Coke (8 oz.) – 100 calories
- Ultra-Light Beer (12 oz.) – 65 to 95 calories
- Mimosa (4 oz.) – 80 calories
- Mike's Hard Lemonade (11 oz.) – 98 calories

Chapter Six: Highest and Lowest Calorie Drinks

<u>If you prefer to engineer your own beverage, try some of these low-calorie mixers:</u>

- Diet Tonic or Soda (8 oz.) – 0 calories
- Orange Juice (6 oz.) – 85 calories
- Cranberry Juice Cocktail (8 oz.) – 135 calories
- Light Lemonade (8 oz.) – 5 calories
- Coffee or Tea (6 oz.) – 0 calories
- Lemon or Lime Juice (1/2 oz.) – 10 calories
- Sugar-Free Syrups (Torani or Davinci) – 0 calories

If you are spending the night at home and still want to enjoy a tasty but low-calorie alcoholic beverage, give some of the recipes in the next chapter a try!

Chapter Seven: Healthy/Low-Calorie Cocktail Choices

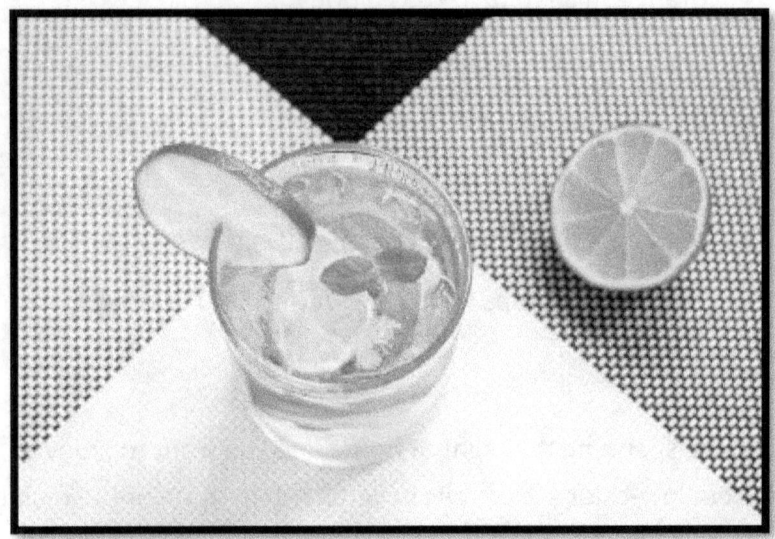

When making your own cocktails at home, you need to be mindful of not only what type of mixer you use but also how much alcohol you add. Even the lowest calorie alcohol – vodka – is still very calorie dense with 7 calories per gram. A 1.5 ounce shot of 80-proof vodka contains 97 calories. If you add a full glass of orange juice or soda, you could be multiplying that calorie count by two or three. To make sure you keep your calorie count down when drinking, try some of the recipes in this chapter.

Chapter Seven: Healthy and Low-Calorie Cocktail Choices

1.) Cocktails Under 200 Calories

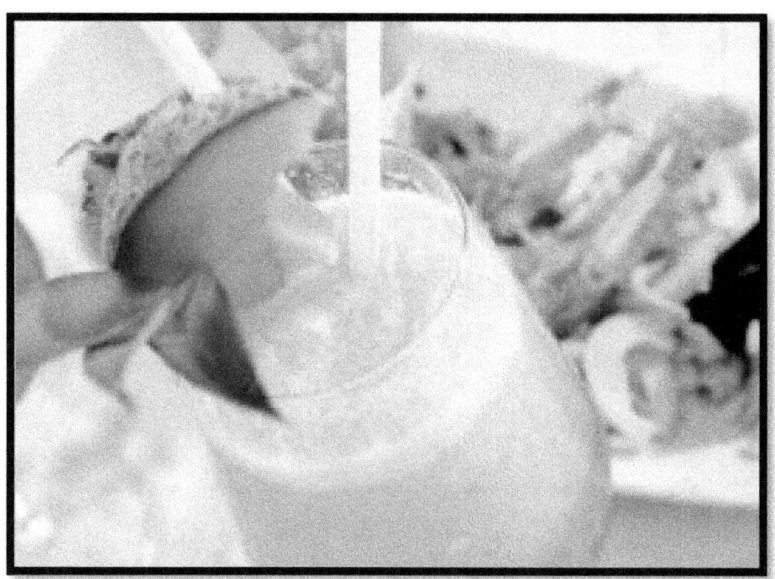

Recipes Included in this Section:

Raspberry Cosmo on Ice	Fresh Mint Mojito
Gin and Tonic - Light	Mulled Wine for a Crowd
Mulled Cider for a Group	Refreshing Sea Breeze
Cucumber Honey Cocktail	Vanilla Cake Cocktail
Hot Toddy	Tequila Soda with Lime
Extra-Light Margarita	Sour Apple Martini

Chapter Seven: Healthy and Low-Calorie Cocktail Choices

Raspberry Cosmo on Ice

Calories: 115 calories

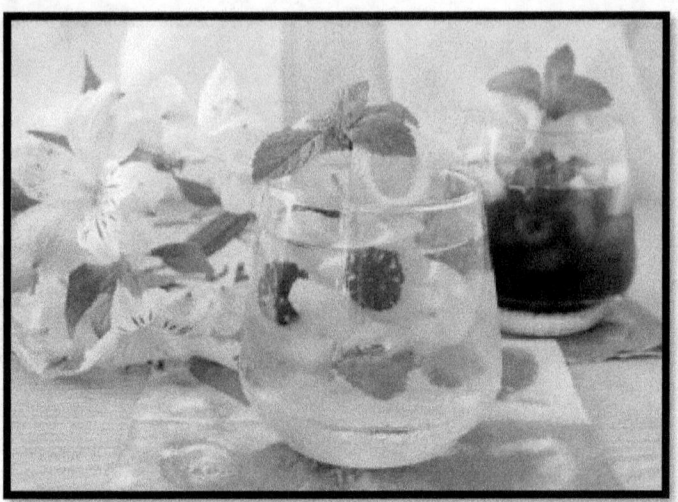

Ingredients:

- 1.5 ounces raspberry vodka
- 6 ounces club soda
- 1 ounce cranberry juice cocktail
- 2 wedges lemon, squeezed

Instructions:

1. Fill a pint glass with ice then pour in the vodka.
2. Add the club soda and top with the cranberry juice cocktail.
3. Squeeze in the lemon then drop the wedges into the glass.

Chapter Seven: Healthy and Low-Calorie Cocktail Choices

Gin and Tonic - Light

Calories: 100 to 140 calories

Ingredients:

- 1 ounce gin
- 1 ounce soda water
- Splash of diet tonic
- Lemon twist

Instructions:

1. Pour the gin and soda water into a metal shaker.
2. Add a scoop of ice and shake until the drink is chilled.
3. Pour the liquid into a large shot glass.
4. Add a splash of tonic and finish with a lemon twist.

Chapter Seven: Healthy and Low-Calorie Cocktail Choices

Mulled Cider for a Group

Calories: 100 calories

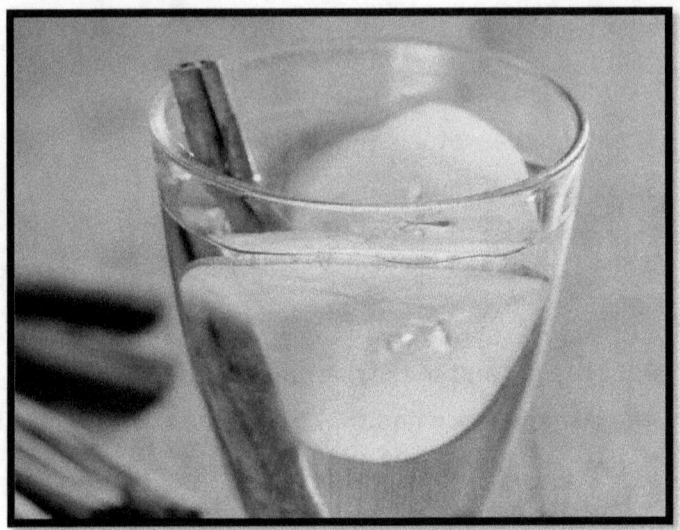

Ingredients:

- 1 gallon apple cider
- 4 cinnamon sticks (2 to 3 inches)
- 1 teaspoon cloves, whole
- 1 teaspoon whole allspice
- 1 ripe apple, cored and sliced
- 1 lemon, sliced
- 1 cup rum

Instructions:

1. Pour the cider into a large saucepan and add the cinnamon, allspice, cloves, apple slices, and lemon.
2. Bring to a boil then reduce heat and simmer, covered, for 45 minutes.

Chapter Seven: Healthy and Low-Calorie Cocktail Choices

3. Stir in the rum and heat through but do not boil.
4. Strain the cider through a mesh sieve into a punch bowl to serve.

Chapter Seven: Healthy and Low-Calorie Cocktail Choices

Cucumber Honey Cocktail

Calories: 135 calories

Ingredients:

- 1 ounce vodka
- 2 slices seedless cucumber, peeled
- 2 ounces green tea, chilled
- ½ ounce fresh lime juice
- 1 tablespoon honey

Instructions:

1. Place the sliced cucumber in a cocktail glass and pour in the vodka.
2. Muddle the cucumber with a pestle then pour in the remaining ingredients.
3. Garnish with a sprig of mint and a lime twist to serve.

Chapter Seven: Healthy and Low-Calorie Cocktail Choices

Hot Toddy

Calories: 115 calories

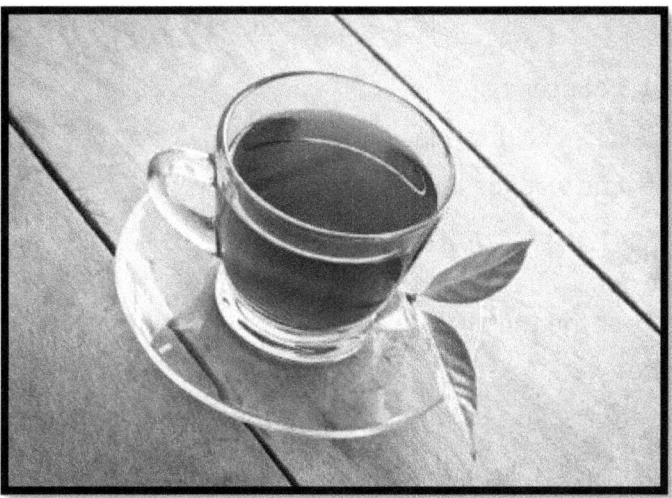

Ingredients:

- 6 ounces hot black tea
- ½ ounce brandy
- 1 tablespoon honey
- 1 tablespoon lemon juice

Instructions:

1. Pour the tea into a coffee mug and add the remaining ingredients.
2. Stir well and serve while hot.

Chapter Seven: Healthy and Low-Calorie Cocktail Choices

Extra-Light Margarita

Calories: 100 calories

Ingredients:

- 1.5 ounces tequila
- Splash of club soda
- 2 lime wedges

Instructions:

1. Pour the tequila into a margarita glass and add a few ice cubes.
2. Add a splash of club soda and squeeze in the lime wedges.
3. Garnish with extra lime and sip slowly.

Chapter Seven: Healthy and Low-Calorie Cocktail Choices

Fresh Mint Mojito

Calories: 150 calories

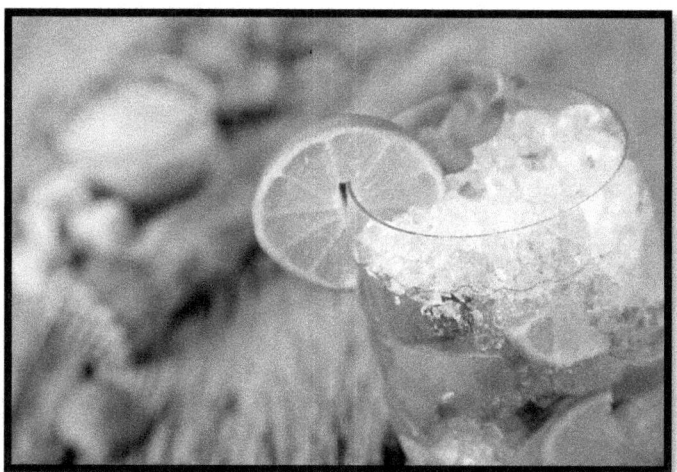

Ingredients:

- 1 shot rum
- 6 ounces soda water
- 2 tablespoons sugar syrup
- 2 lime wedges
- 1 tablespoon fresh mint

Instructions:

1. Place the mint in a cocktail glass and add the rum.
2. Muddle the mint with a pestle then add the remaining ingredients.
3. Stir well and serve immediately.

Mulled Wine for a Crowd

Calories: 130 calories

Ingredients:

- 6 to 8 cloves
- 4 whole peppercorns
- 2 tablespoons lemon zest
- 2 tablespoons orange zest
- 4 cups dry red wine
- 1 ½ cups water
- ½ cup cherry-flavored brandy
- 2/3 cup raw cane sugar
- 1 cinnamon stick (2 to 3 inches)
- 1 vanilla bean, halved

Instructions:

1. Place the cloves, peppercorns, lemon zest, and orange zest in a small mesh pouch.
2. Pour the red wine, water, brandy, and sugar in a saucepot.
3. Add the mesh pouch along with the cinnamon stick and vanilla bean.
4. Bring to a boil then simmer for 10 minutes before serving.

Chapter Seven: Healthy and Low-Calorie Cocktail Choices

Refreshing Sea Breeze

Calories: 175 calories

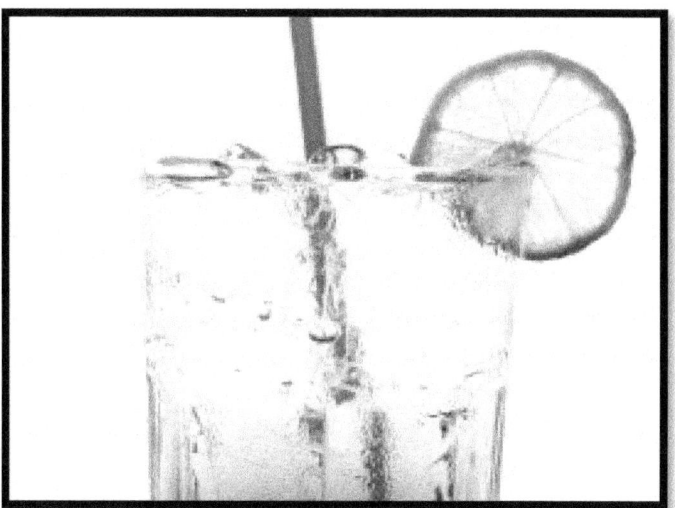

Ingredients:

- 4 ounces grapefruit juice
- 1 ½ ounces cranberry juice cocktail
- 1 ounce vodka

Instructions:

1. Fill a tall glass with ice.
2. Add the remaining ingredients and stir well.
3. Garnish with an orange wedge to serve.

Chapter Seven: Healthy and Low-Calorie Cocktail Choices

Vanilla Cake Cocktail

Calories: 90 calories

Ingredients:

- 1 shot vanilla vodka
- 6 ounces diet ginger ale

Instructions:

1. Pour the vodka into a cocktail glass and add ice.
2. Add the ginger ale and serve with a lemon twist.

Chapter Seven: Healthy and Low-Calorie Cocktail Choices

Tequila Soda with Lime

Calories: 100 calories

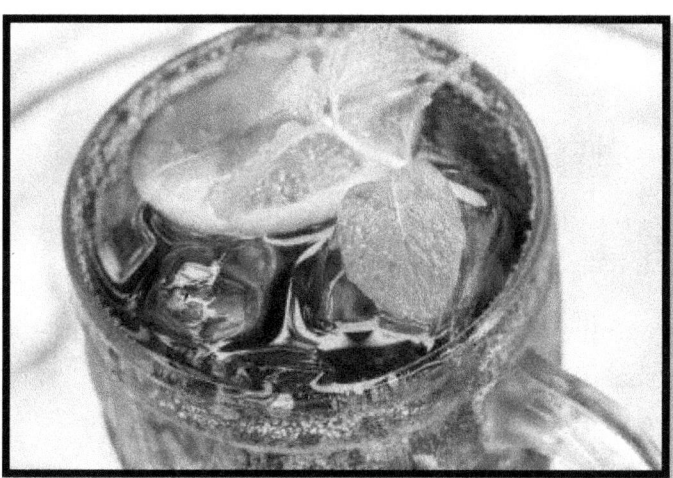

Ingredients:

- 1 shot tequila
- 6 ounces diet soda or club soda
- 2 lime wedges

Instructions:

1. Fill a short glass with ice cubes.
2. Add the tequila and fill the glass with diet soda or club soda.
3. Squeeze in a lime wedge and garnish with extra lime to serve.

Chapter Seven: Healthy and Low-Calorie Cocktail Choices

Sour Apple Martini

Calories: 155 calories

Ingredients:

- 2 ½ ounces sour mix
- ¾ ounces vodka
- ¾ ounce sour apple liqueur

Instructions:

1. Combine the sour mix, vodka and liqueur in a metal shaker.
2. Add ice and shake until chilled.
3. Strain the liquid in a chilled martini glass.
4. Garnish with a slice of apple to serve.

Chapter Seven: Healthy and Low-Calorie Cocktail Choices

2.) Healthy Cocktails with Fruit

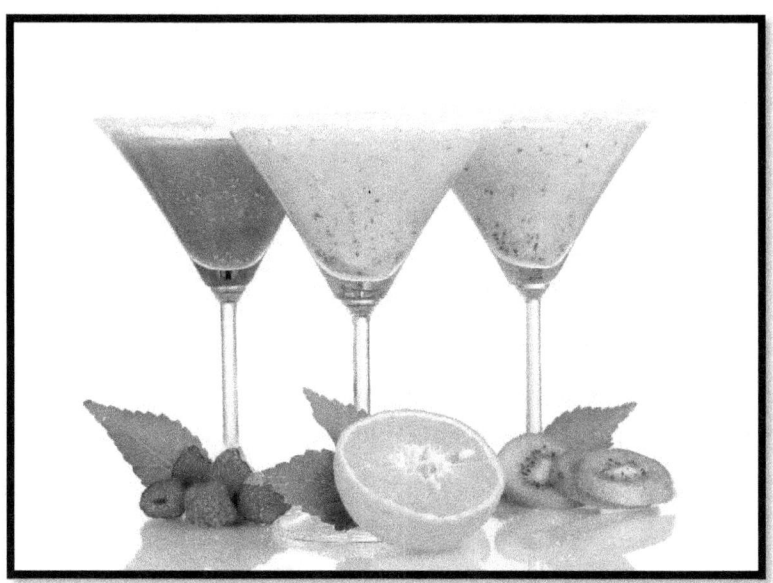

Recipes Included in this Section:

Frozen Blueberry Margarita	Orange Old Fashioned
Sweet Tropical Limeade	Kiwi Tom Collins
Gin and Watermelon Fizz	Pineapple Champagne Cooler
Refreshing Blueberry Bellini	Spicy Grapefruit Margarita
Blackberry Coconut Daiquiri	Lemon Gin Fizz with Rosemary
Bloody Mary	Watermelon Sunrise
Raspberry Mojito	Honeydew Sparklers
Strawberry Coconut Margarita	Melon Sangria
Razzy Pink Cosmo	Mint Strawberry Mojito

Chapter Seven: Healthy and Low-Calorie Cocktail Choices

Frozen Blueberry Margarita

Blueberries are one of the highest food sources of antioxidants. Antioxidants help to protect your body against free-radical damage and they may also help to reduce your risk for certain types of cancer.

Calories: 130 calories

Ingredients:

- 1 cup ice cubes
- ½ cup frozen blueberries
- ½ cup blueberry nectar
- 2 tablespoons club soda
- 1 tablespoon fresh lime juice
- 1.5 ounce shot tequila
- Lime wedge

Instructions:

1. Combine all of the ingredients except the lime wedge in a high-speed blender.
2. Blend on high speed for 30 to 45 seconds until smooth and well combined.
3. Use the lime wedge to wet the rim of a martini glass and dip it in salt.
4. Pour the margarita into the glass and drop in the lime wedge.

Chapter Seven: Healthy and Low-Calorie Cocktail Choices

Sweet Tropical Limeade

Lime has been known to provide a number of significant health benefits including improved digestion, rejuvenated skin, and reduced risk for constipation. Limes also contain special compounds called flavonoids which provide detoxification, antioxidant, and anti-carcinogenic benefits for the body.

Calories: 170 calories

Ingredients:

- 3 cups hot water
- ½ cup 1 tbsp raw cane sugar
- 1 ¼ cups fresh lime juice
- 4 shots dark rum
- 2 limes, sliced thin

Instructions:

1. Bring the water and sugar to boil in a saucepan, stirring until the sugar has dissolved.
2. Remove from heat and stir in the lime juice – let cool for 10 minutes.
3. Fill four glasses with ice and thin slices of lime.
4. Add 1 shot of dark rum to each glass and fill the rest of the way with the limeade.

Chapter Seven: Healthy and Low-Calorie Cocktail Choices

Gin and Watermelon Fizz

Watermelon consists of about 92% water which makes it excellent for combating dehydration. This fruit also contains high levels of a variety of nutrients including vitamin A, vitamin C, lycopene, antioxidants, and various amino acids.

Calories: 150 calories

Ingredients:

- 4 cups seedless watermelon, chopped
- 6 ounces gin, divided
- 1 cup fresh lime juice, divided
- 2 cups ginger ale, divided
- 4 lime wedges

Instructions:

1. Fill four tall glasses with ice.
2. Place the watermelon in a food processor and puree until smooth.
3. Strain the watermelon through a mesh sieve and divide the liquid among the four glasses.
4. Add a 1.5 ounce shot of gin to each glass along with 2 tablespoons of lime juice and 3 to 4 ounces of ginger ale.
5. Garnish with a lime wedge to serve.

Chapter Seven: Healthy and Low-Calorie Cocktail Choices

Refreshing Blueberry Bellini

In addition to being rich in antioxidants, blueberries are also loaded with healthy nutrients. Blueberries are an excellent source of vitamins including vitamin A, B, E and C as well as minerals like zinc, selenium, and iron.

Calories: 180 calories

Ingredients:

- ½ cup fresh blueberries
- 2 tablespoons fresh lemon juice
- Pinch ground ginger
- 2 cups fresh blueberry juice, unsweetened
- 2 cups sparkling wine

Instructions:

1. Combine the blueberries, sugar, lemon juice and ginger in a mixing bowl.
2. Mash the berries with the other ingredients using the back of a wooden spoon.
3. Stir in the blueberry juice and let rest for 5 minutes.
4. Strain the mixture and divide the liquid among four wine glasses or champagne flutes.
5. Pour 4 ounces of sparkling wine into each glass to serve.

Chapter Seven: Healthy and Low-Calorie Cocktail Choices

Blackberry Coconut Daiquiri

Fresh blackberries provide excellent digestive and cardiovascular benefits due to their high fiber content. A single cup of blackberries contains 8 grams of fiber which is about 30% of your daily recommended allotment. Blackberries are also rich in vitamin K which is essential for bone health.

Calories: 115 calories

Ingredients:

- 2 ½ cups frozen blackberries
- 1 tbsp raw cane sugar
- 2 tablespoons fresh lime juice
- 3 cups ice cubes, crushed
- 6 ounces Malibu rum

Instructions:

1. Place the blackberries, sugar, and lime juice in a high-speed blender.
2. Blend on high speed for 30 to 60 seconds until smooth.
3. Add the ice cubes and rum then blend until slushy.
4. Divide the mixture among short cocktail glasses – makes about 10 servings.

Chapter Seven: Healthy and Low-Calorie Cocktail Choices

Bloody Mary

Tomatoes are naturally loaded with healthy vitamins and minerals. Not only are they low in calories and rich in vitamin C, but they also contain beta-carotene which can help to improve the health of your skin – it also helps to protect your skin against sun damage.

Calories: 120 calories

Ingredients:

- 1 ¼ cups chilled tomato juice
- 2 ounces vodka
- 1 tablespoon hot sauce
- 1 tablespoon Worcestershire sauce
- 4 pitted green olives
- 2 small stalks celery

Instructions:

1. Combine the tomato juice, vodka, hot sauce, and Worcestershire sauce in a mixing bowl.
2. Stir well then divide between the two glasses.
3. Add two olives and a stalk of celery to each glass to finish.

Chapter Seven: Healthy and Low-Calorie Cocktail Choices

Raspberry Mojito

Fresh raspberries are loaded with vitamins and nutrients. A single cup of raspberries contains 8 grams dietary fiber and 1.5 grams protein – they are also rich in calcium, lutein, vitamin C, and a variety of other antioxidants.

Calories: 160 calories

Ingredients:

- 4 to 6 fresh blackberries
- 1 tablespoon fresh mint leaves
- 2 ounces vodka
- 1 teaspoon sugar
- 4 ounces diet club soda
- 1 ounce fresh lime juice

Instructions:

1. Place the blackberries and mint in a tall glass.
2. Muddle the fruit and mint with a pestle or spoon then fill the glass with ice.
3. Combine the vodka, sugar, club soda and lime juice in a metal shaker.
4. Add ice and shake until chilled.
5. Strain the liquid into the cocktail glass and serve.

Chapter Seven: Healthy and Low-Calorie Cocktail Choices

Strawberry Coconut Margarita

Strawberries are incredibly rich in vitamin C, a vitamin that is essential for immune system health. A single serving of strawberries contains about 51 mg of vitamin C which is about 50% of your daily recommended allotment.

Calories: 120 calories

Ingredients:

- 2 ½ cups frozen sliced strawberries
- 1 -2 tbsp raw cane sugar
- 2 tablespoons fresh lime juice
- 3 cups ice cubes
- 6 ounces tequila
- 1 ounce Malibu rum

Instructions:

1. Place the strawberries, sugar, and lime juice in a high-speed blender.
2. Blend on high speed for 30 to 60 seconds until smooth.
3. Add the ice cubes, tequila and rum then blend until slushy.
4. Divide the mixture among margarita glasses – makes about 10 servings.

Chapter Seven: Healthy and Low-Calorie Cocktail Choices

Razzy Pink Cosmo

This tasty cocktail combines the flavors of raspberry and lime. Lime is very rich in vitamin C and it provides natural antibiotic, antioxidant, and anti-cancer benefits.

Calories: 260

Ingredients:

- 1 cup frozen raspberries
- ¾ cups water
- 2 ounces vodka
- 1 ounce raspberry liqueur
- 1 tablespoon fresh lime juice

Instructions:

1. Combine the frozen raspberries and water in a small saucepan and bring to a simmer.
2. Mash the berries with a spoon then strain the liquid into a cup, pressing on the berries to release their juice.
3. Pour 1 ounce of the raspberry juice into a shaker with the vodka, raspberry liquor and lime juice.
4. Add ice and shake until very cold then pour into a chilled martini glass.
5. Garnish with fresh or frozen raspberries, if desired.

Chapter Seven: Healthy and Low-Calorie Cocktail Choices

Orange Old Fashioned

Not only are oranges known for their fresh, flavorful juice but they are also packed with healthy nutrients. Oranges are rich in vitamin C which can boost your immune system and improve your skin and heart health.

Calories: 245

Ingredients:

- 1 tbsp raw cane sugar
- 1 teaspoon bitters
- 1 navel orange
- 2 ounces bourbon whiskey
- 2 maraschino cherries

Instructions:

1. Cut the orange in half and juice one half then cut the other half into wedges.
2. Combine the sugar and bitters in a short glass and muddle with a spoon.
3. Pour in a few tablespoons of orange juice and muddle again.
4. Add a few ice cubes and top it off with the bourbon.
5. Garnish with a few maraschino cherries and an orange wedge to serve.

Chapter Seven: Healthy and Low-Calorie Cocktail Choices

Kiwi Tom Collins

In addition to being loaded with flavor, fresh kiwi is also an excellent source of dietary fiber which helps to support healthy digestion. Kiwifruit is also low in calories but rich in vitamin C and potassium.

Calories: 245

Ingredients:

- 1 ripe kiwi, peeled and chopped
- 2 fresh mint leaves
- 2 ounces gin
- 1 ounce simple syrup
- 2 tablespoons fresh lime juice
- Splash club soda

Instructions:

1. Combine the kiwi and mint in a small bowl and mash them together with a fork or spoon.
2. Transfer the kiwi mint mixture to a Tom Collins glass and add ice cubes.
3. Combine the gin, lime juice, and simple syrup in a shaker with ice and shake until cold.
4. Pour the mixture into your glass and top it off with a splash of club soda.

Chapter Seven: Healthy and Low-Calorie Cocktail Choices

Tropical Pineapple Champagne Cooler

Fresh pineapple is an excellent source of vitamins and minerals. A single 1-cup serving contains more than 100% your daily value for vitamin C as well as plenty of calcium, iron, magnesium and potassium. It is also rich in polyphenols and antioxidants.

Calories: 130

Ingredients:

- 1 ½ ounces pineapple juice
- 1 ½ ounces coconut juice or coconut water
- Chilled champagne

Instructions:

1. Pour the pineapple juice and coconut juice into a champagne flute.
2. Fill the glass the rest of the way with champagne and serve immediately.
3. To decorate the glasses, dip the rims in simple syrup then in shredded coconut before adding the liquid.

Chapter Seven: Healthy and Low-Calorie Cocktail Choices

Spicy Grapefruit Margarita

Grapefruit is a good source of dietary fiber as well as vitamins and minerals like calcium, magnesium, vitamin A and vitamin C. It is also a low-calorie food which can help to promote weight loss.

Calories: 240

Ingredients:

- 2 slices fresh grapefruit
- 1/8 teaspoon juice from canned chipotle peppers
- 2 tablespoons fresh lime juice
- 1 ounce simple syrup
- 1.5 ounces tequila
- ½ ounce triple sec

Instructions:

1. Dip the rim of a glass drinking jar in simple syrup then in salt to coat.
2. Place the grapefruit and chipotle juice in a cocktail shaker and muddle with the lime juice.
3. Add the simple syrup, triple sec, and tequila then shake with ice until cold.
4. Fill the glass jar with ice and strain the liquid over it.
5. Garnish with a slice of grapefruit to serve.

Chapter Seven: Healthy and Low-Calorie Cocktail Choices

Lemon Gin Fizz with Rosemary

This cocktail combines the flavors and health benefits of lemon and rosemary. Lemon is a great food for detoxing and rosemary is loaded with antioxidants and anti-inflammatory compounds. Rosemary can also help protect your brain against neurodegenerative disease.

Calories: 175

Ingredients:

- 1 cup water
- 1 tbsp raw cane sugar
- 1 sprig rosemary
- 1 strip lemon zest (2 inches)
- 2 ounces gin
- 1 ½ ounces fresh lemon juice
- Splash club soda
- Lemon wedge

Instructions:

1. Combine the water, rosemary, sugar and lemon zest in a small saucepan.
2. Bring the mixture to a simmer and simmer for 2 minutes.
3. Remove from heat and let rest for 15 minutes then strain the liquid into a glass and chill.
4. Fill a cocktail shaker with ice then add the gin, lemon juice, and ¾ ounces of the rosemary syrup.
5. Shake until cold then pour into a highball glass filled with ice.
6. Top the glass off with a splash of club soda and garnish with a lemon wedge.

Chapter Seven: Healthy and Low-Calorie Cocktail Choices

Watermelon Sunrise

This watermelon sunrise is the perfect drink to serve your guests on a hot summer day. Not only is it thirst-quenching and refreshing, but it is loaded with antioxidants and healthy vitamins.

Calories: 155

Ingredients:

- ¼ cup water
- 1 tbsp raw cane sugar
- 1 lbs. seedless watermelon, chopped
- Juice from 2 limes
- 1 ½ cups fresh raspberries
- ½ cup fresh mint leaves
- 1 ¼ cups tequila

Instructions:

1. Combine the water and sugar in a small saucepan and bring to a simmer to make the simple syrup.
2. Simmer for 1 minute until the sugar is dissolved then set aside to cool.
3. Place the watermelon in a blender and blend until pureed then strain it over a bowl to collect the juice.
4. Combine the simple syrup and lime juice in a glass pitcher with the raspberries and mint.
5. Gently muddle the berries using a wooden spoon then stir in the watermelon juice and tequila.
6. Chill for 2 hours before pouring into glasses over ice to serve. Garnish with mint.

Chapter Seven: Healthy and Low-Calorie Cocktail Choices

Honeydew Sparklers

Honeydew is a type of melon and it is loaded with both vitamin A and vitamin C. Additionally, honeydew is low in calories and rich in nutrients that help to reduce cholesterol, improve bone and tooth strength, and aid healthy digestion.

Calories: 245

Ingredients:

1 (3 to 3 ½ lbs.) honeydew, peeled and seeded

1 (750 ml.) bottle sweet white wine

Champagne

Instructions:

1. Use a melon baller to scoop about 2 cups of honeydew then chop the remaining fruit.
2. Place the chopped honeydew in a blender and blend until smooth then strain through a sieve, pressing out as much moisture as possible.
3. In a small saucepan, bring the wine to boil then simmer until reduced to about 2 tablespoons, about 10 minutes.
4. Add the reduced wine to the honeydew juice and stir well.
5. Fill champagne flutes with the balled honeydew then add champagne until filled within 1 inch of the top.
6. Top each glass off with a splash of the melon juice mixture.

Melon Sangria

While the exact benefits of different types of melon vary, they are all right in essential vitamins and minerals as well as sweet, juicy flavor. This melon sangria is loaded with vitamin C, vitamin A, and potassium as well as other nutrients.

Calories: 230

Ingredients:

- 2 cups seedless watermelon, chopped
- 2 cups chopped cantaloupe, seeded
- 2 cups chopped honeydew, seeded
- 1 bottle white wine, dry
- 2/3 cup vodka
- ½ cup triple sec
- ½ cup simple syrup

Instructions:

1. Place the watermelon, cantaloupe and honeydew in a blender and blend until pureed.
2. Strain the liquid through a strainer, pressing on the pulp to release as much juice as possible.
3. Pour the liquid into a pitcher and add the wine, vodka, triple sec and simple syrup.
4. Stir well and chill for 2 hours.
5. Pour the sangria into short glasses filled with ice.

Chapter Seven: Healthy and Low-Calorie Cocktail Choices

Mint Strawberry Mojito

Mint is an herb that is known not only for its fresh flavor but also for the many health benefits it provides. This herb soothes upset stomach and relieves headache – it can also relieve respiratory problems including cough and asthma.

Calories: 170

Ingredients:

- 2 fresh strawberries, diced
- 12 leaves fresh mint
- 2 lemon wedges
- 2 ounces rum
- 1 tablespoon fresh lemon juice
- ½ ounce simple syrup

Instructions:

1. Combine the strawberries and mint in a cocktail shaker and muddle gently with a spoon.
2. Add the lemon wedges, rum, lemon juice and simple syrup then fill the shaker with ice.
3. Shake until the liquid is very cold then strain over a highball glass filled with ice.

Resources

"5 Sneaky Ways Alcohol Affects Your Health and Beauty." TotalBeauty.com. <http://www.totalbeauty.com/content/gallery/alcohol-makes-you-ugly/p82952/page2>

Aaron, Kiera. "Why You Eat When You're Drunk." Men's Health. <http://www.menshealth.com/mhu/food/why-you-eat-when-youre-drunk>

"Abdominal Obesity and Your Health." The Harvard Medical School Family Health Guide. <http://www.health.harvard.edu/fhg/updates/abdominal-obesity-and-your-health.shtml>

"Absorption Rate Factors." McDonald Center for Student Well-Being. <http://oade.nd.edu/educate-yourself-alcohol/absorbtion-rate-factors/>

"Alcohol and Nutrition." MedicineNet.com. <http://www.medicinenet.com/alcohol_and_nutrition/page4.htm>

Resources

Ansel, Karen. "Drinking Alcohol to Shrink?" Women's Health Magazine Online. <http://www.womenshealthmag.com/weight-loss/alcohol-drinking-and-weight-loss-tips>

Bryan, Adam. "Gluten Free Alcohol List." Munchyy.com. <http://munchyy.com/gluten-free-alcohol-list/>

"Effect of Drugs and Alcohol on the Immune System." AlcoholRehab.com. <http://alcoholrehab.com/drug-addiction/drugs-alcohol-immune-system/>

Goins, Liesa. "How to Hold Your Liquor." WebMD. <http://www.webmd.com/balance/features/how-to-hold-your-liquor?page=1>

Greenspan, Sam. "11 Best Beers to Get You Drunk But Not Make You Fat." 11 Points. <http://www.11points.com/Food-Drink/11_Best_Beers_To_Get_You_Drunk_But_Not_Make_You_Fat>

Hanson, Prof. David J. "Alcohol 'Proof' and 'Alcohol by Volume': Definitions and Explanations." State University of New York, Sociology Department. <http://www2.potsdam.edu/alcohol/StateAndLocalLaws/20070531155139.html#.VLVKEyvF9DQ>

Resources

"How to Drink Without Gaining Weight." Health.com. <http://www.health.com/health/article/0,,20670897,00.html>

"How Much Sleep Do We Really Need?" National Sleep Foundation. < http://sleepfoundation.org/how-sleep-works/how-much-sleep-do-we-really-need>

Hyman, Mark. "Three Hidden Ways Wheat Makes You Fat." DrHyman.com. <http://drhyman.com/blog/2012/02/13/three-hidden-ways-wheat-makes-you-fat/#close>

Ingraham, Christopher. "The Wonkblog Guide to Efficient Drinking." The Washington Post. <http://www.washingtonpost.com/blogs/wonkblog/wp/2014/03/28/the-wonkblog-guide-to-efficient-drinking/>

"Is Alcohol an Endocrine Disruptor?" Global Healing Center. <http://www.globalhealingcenter.com/natural-health/is-alcohol-an-endocrine-disruptor/>

"Is It Possible to Drink and Still be Healthy?" Nerd Fitness Blog. <http://www.nerdfitness.com/blog/2012/05/10/alcohol/>

Resources

"Low-Calorie Cocktails." WebMD. <http://www.webmd.com/diet/features/low-calorie-cocktails?page=1>

"Taking a Break from Alcohol: Suggestions for 30 Days." McDonald Center for Student Well-Being. <http://oade.nd.edu/educate-yourself-alcohol/taking-a-break-from-alcohol-suggestions-for-30-days/>

"The 9 Worst Cocktails for Weight Loss." Fitness Magazine. <http://www.fitnessmagazine.com/weight-loss/eating-help/calories/worst-cocktails/?page=9>

"The Importance of Water and Your Health." FreeDrinkingWater.com. <http://www.freedrinkingwater.com/water-education/water-health.htm>

"The Ten Most Fattening Cocktails." Forbes.com. <http://www.forbes.com/2006/12/06/fattening-drinks-cocktails-forbeslife-cx_1207cocktails_slide.html>

"Your Body and Alcohol." McDonald Center for Student Well-Being. <http://oade.nd.edu/educate-yourself-alcohol/your-body-and-alcohol/>

Resources

"What Causes Beer Belly?" BBC Future. <http://www.bbc.com/future/story/20130920-what-causes-a-beer-belly>

"Why Does Drinking Cause Dehydration?" ABC Science. <http://www.abc.net.au/science/articles/2012/02/28/3441707.htm>

Zelman, Kathleen. "The Truth About Beer and Your Belly." WebMD. < http://www.webmd.com/diet/features/the-truth-about-beer-and-your-belly?page=1>

Index

A

abdominal obesity 22, 23, 25
absorption 18, 34, 40, 41, 42, 43, 44, 46, 47, 49, 51, 52
ABV 5, 6, 7, 8, 10, 11, 12, 13, 14
addiction 39, 46, 105
ADH 17
agave 28
aging 15, 16, 17
alcohol 3, 2, 3, 4, 5, 6, 7, 8, 9, 10, 11, 13, 14, 15, 16, 17, 18, 20, 21, 22, 23, 26, 27, 29, 33, 34, 35, 36, 37, 38, 39, 40, 41, 42, 43, 44, 46, 47, 51, 52, 64, 65, 70, 104, 105, 106, 107
Alcohol by volume 5
alcoholic hepatitis 39
anti-diuretic hormone 17
anxiety 37, 65
appearance 23

B

BAC 41, 43, 44, 45, 46, 47, 64
beer 1, 5, 7, 9, 11, 12, 13, 16, 22, 23, 25, 27, 29, 108
beer belly 22, 23
blood 17, 19, 32, 34, 36, 38, 39, 41, 42, 51, 52, 54
Blood Alcohol Concentration 41
blurred vision 33, 37, 38
body ... 3, 2, 3, 6, 7, 8, 15, 16, 17, 18, 21, 22, 23, 24, 31, 32, 33, 34, 35, 36, 37, 38, 40, 41, 43, 46, 47, 49, 51, 52, 53, 64, 107
body image 7
body temperature 32
bones 32
brain 25, 32, 36, 37
brands 26, 27, 28
brandy 6
breathalyzer 38

Index

build muscle 7
buzz 3, 2, 3, 4, 5, 8, 9, 10, 12, 13, 14, 40, 41

C

calorie content 2, 3, 10, 66
calories 3, 1, 3, 4, 5, 7, 10, 12, 13, 18, 20, 21, 22, 23, 29, 30, 42, 45, 51, 66, 67, 68, 69, 70, 107
cancer 17, 33
carbohydrates 18, 42
carbs 1, 7, 38, 45, 52
central nervous system 37
club soda 14, 50
cocktails 45, 52, 66, 67, 68, 70, 107
coordination 37
cravings 16, 18, 26, 45, 66

D

dehydration 15, 33
dehydrogenase 43
depression 65
designated driver 8
dessert wine 6
diabetes 19, 24, 26
diarrhea 25
diet 8, 14, 21, 107, 108
digestion 32
disease 17, 19, 24, 25, 26, 27, 39
distillation 27
distilled liquors 4, 10, 14
doctor 47, 65

E

effects 2, 3, 15, 16, 17, 18, 36, 37, 38, 39, 46, 47, 50, 51, 52
electrolyte balance 17

Index

endocrine system	18
energy	18, 22, 38
enzymes	32, 46
ethanol	4, 5, 18
exercise	8, 21, 54

F

family history	64

fat 6, 7, 21, 22, 23, 24, 42, 43, 52, 57, 61, 63, 106

fatigue	25, 31, 33, 53
fluid balance	34
fluids	16
food	18, 19, 22, 26, 31, 32, 40, 41, 42, 45, 52, 66, 104
frequency	39, 64, 65
fruit juice	34, 49
functional tolerance	46, 64

G

gin 6, 10

glucose	18, 38
gluten	25, 26, 27, 28, 29, 105
gluten sensitivity	25, 27
gluten-free	26, 27, 28, 29, 105
glycogen	19
goals	3, 1, 2, 3, 5, 6, 7, 8, 9, 10, 26, 48, 51, 54, 64

H

hangover	33, 34, 49
hard cider	27
headache	25, 33
healing	39
healthy	2, 7, 8, 18, 42, 44, 49, 52, 53, 64
heart attack	24
HGH	38

Index

hormone regulation 16
hormones 18, 19
human growth hormone 38
hydrated 17, 32, 33, 42, 49

I

immune system 15, 16, 17
inflammation 39
insulin 16, 18, 38
intestinal tract 17, 49
intoxication 40
IPA 11, 12, 13, 14

J

joints 32
judgment 38, 64

K

kidneys 17, 53

L

leaky gut syndrome 49
lifestyle 7, 35
lightweight 46
liver 17, 18, 19, 23, 38, 39, 41, 50, 53
long-term 15, 18, 19, 39
low-calorie 2, 7, 8, 14, 50, 66, 69, 107
lubricant 32

Index

M

medications	46, 47
memories	36
men	23, 24, 39, 40, 43
metabolic syndrome	24
metabolism	18, 22, 23, 54
mixed drinks	42
mixers	34, 49, 69
mood	18, 40, 46

N

nausea	65
non-alcoholic	8, 34, 49
nutrients	16, 17, 18, 33, 49, 53
nutrition	38, 53, 104
nutritional deficiency	17

O

organs	17, 32, 53
osteoporosis	18

P

pain	25, 33, 37, 47
pancreatitis	39
perspiration	32, 65
prescriptions	47
proof	4, 5, 70
protein	7, 25, 27, 38, 42, 52, 57

R

recipes	4, 2, 69, 70

Index

rehydrate 34, 53
rum 6, 10, 34

S

sake 6
serving size 11, 13
short-term 15, 16
sick 47
skin 17, 32
sleep 8, 35, 36, 38, 106
slurred speech 37
sober 52
sparkling wine 14
sports drink 34
strength training 7
stress 1, 37
stroke 24
sweating 32, 38

T

tequila 6, 28
tips 2, 7, 12, 48, 49, 105
tolerance 46, 64

U

ulcers 18
urinate 16, 17

V

vitamins 18
vodka 6, 10, 70

Index

W

waist circumference 24
waist-to-hip ratio 24
water 16, 17, 31, 32, 33, 34, 39, 42, 43, 49, 51, 53, 107
water-soluble 33
weight . 3, 1, 2, 3, 4, 6, 7, 9, 10, 16, 20, 23, 26, 43, 45, 48, 49, 51, 54, 64, 66, 67, 105, 107
weight loss 2, 3, 26, 51, 54, 64
wheat 25, 27, 106
whisky 6, 11
wine 1, 4, 5, 7, 10, 11, 13, 14, 21, 34, 39
women 20, 21, 23, 24, 39, 40, 43
workout 38